The Doc[...]
Tale

Professionalism and public trust

Donald Irvine
Immediate Past President
General Medical Council

Radcliffe Medical Press

Radcliffe Medical Press Ltd
18 Marcham Road
Abingdon
Oxon OX14 1AA
United Kingdom

www.radcliffe-oxford.com
The Radcliffe Medical Press electronic catalogue and online ordering facility.
Direct sales to anywhere in the world.

British Library Cataloguing in Publication Data

A catalogue record for this book is available from the British Library.

ISBN 1 85775 977 X

Typeset by Joshua Associates Ltd, Oxford
Printed and bound by TJ International Ltd, Padstow, Cornwall

Contents

This book represents the author's interpretation of events against a background of the organisations, culture and individuals that have influenced them. They include men and women who have given long and honourable service to their professions and patients in their care.

Inevitably, some readers may see these events from a different perspective, and interpret them differently. Inevitably, some of the individuals featured in the book may feel they have been misrepresented. This is a personal account and any offence which may be caused is certainly unintended and regretted.

However, subjective interpretation is an entitlement of us all and neither the author, nor the publisher, will accept liability to those who may challenge this account.

Acknowledgements

As I gathered my thoughts together for this book, I had most helpful conversations with many people – patients, doctors, politicians, civil servants and others. I am most grateful for the time, the valuable advice and insights they gave.

Special thanks go to a number of good friends – Rosemary Day, Liam Donaldson, Ruth Evans, Denis Pereira Gray, David Shaw, Catherine Swarbrick and William Wells – who had the burdensome task of looking at an early manuscript. Steve Dewar, Rosalind Foster, Andrew Pugh and Marshall Marinker were kind enough to comment on individual chapters. They all took immense trouble, and gave exactly the kind of robust criticism and honest advice that I needed.

Isabel Nisbet, Finlay Scott and Jane O'Brien, all staff of the GMC, made sure as far as they could that I got my facts right and gave me very good advice. I am most grateful to them. Any errors that remain are entirely my responsibility.

My thanks to Anne Whensley who, as ever, performed miracles in producing drafts in impossible timescales.

Gill Nineham, Jamie Etherington and Gregory Moxon at Radcliffe Medical Press have given enormous support and encouragement, and have shown great patience and flexibility.

My wife, Sally, to whom this book is dedicated, has been terrific throughout. Only she and I know what the enterprise has involved.

List of abbreviations

APD	Accredited Professional Development
AVMA	Action for Victims of Medical Accidents
AVSD	atrio ventricular septal defects
BMA	British Medical Association
BMJ	*British Medical Journal*
BRI	Bristol Royal Infirmary
CA	Consumers' Association
CCSC	Central Consultants' and Specialists' Committee
CCST	Certificate of Completion of Specialist Training
CHAI	Commission for Health Audit and Inspection
CHI	Commission for Health Improvement
CMO	Chief Medical Officer
CNO	Chief Nursing Officer
CPD	Continuing Professional Development
CRHP	Council for the Regulation of Health Professionals
DoH	Department of Health
EEC	European Economic Community
FBA	Fellowship by Assessment [of the Royal College of General Practitioners]
FPC	Family Practitioner Committee
GMC	General Medical Council
GMSC	General Medical Services Committee
GPC	General Practitioners' Committee
JCC	Joint Consultants' Committee
JCPTGP	Joint Committee on Postgraduate Training for General Practitioners
LMC	Local Medical Committee
MAAG	Medical Audit Advisory Group
MRCGP	membership examination of the Royal College of General Practitioners
NCAA	National Clinical Assessment Authority
NCC	National Consumer Council

NHS	National Health Service
NICE	National Institute for Clinical Excellence
NPSA	National Patient Safety Agency
NSF	National Service Framework
PAC	President's Advisory Committee
PCC	Professional Conduct Committee
PGEA	Postgraduate Education Allowance
PMS	Personal Medical Services
PPC	Preliminary Proceedings Committee
RCGP	Royal College of General Practitioners
RCOG	Royal College of Obstetricians and Gynaecologists
RCP	Royal College of Physicians [of London]
RCS	Royal College of Surgeons [of London]
RSM	Royal Society of Medicine
SIGN	Scottish Intercollegiate Guidelines Network
SPM	serious professional misconduct
STA	Specialist Training Authority
UBHT	United Bristol Healthcare NHS Trust
UKCC	United Kingdom Council for Nursing, Midwifery and Health Visiting

For Sally.

Prologue

Bristol: the beginning, the middle or the end?

On 18 June 1998 the council chamber of the General Medical Council (GMC) was packed. The boxes of evidence were piled high. The lawyers looked serious and expectant. The press and public galleries were full to overflowing, journalists elbowing each other to get the best view of the drama unfolding below. As I led the Conduct Committee members back into the chamber, a hush fell. The Bristol drama was reaching its climax, its denouement. I glanced down at my papers to check the words I was about to use, and then looked up into the sea of faces. The atmosphere was electric – you could hear a pin drop. I was all too aware of the significance of what I was about to say, and what it could mean for the future relationships between the public and doctors. Three doctors, the distressed families of deceased or damaged children, concerned friends and colleagues, an embarrassed and troubled profession, an expectant press and a worried public were waiting to hear our decisions.

James Wisheart, a cardiac surgeon, and John Roylance, a medically qualified hospital manager, were found guilty of serious professional misconduct (SPM), and were erased from the Medical Register. Janardan Dhasmana, another heart surgeon, was also found guilty of SPM. In his case the Committee decided that there were mitigating circumstances and stopped him from practising paediatric cardiac surgery for three years, after which the situation would be reviewed.

The GMC's 'Bristol Case', as it has become known, involved the practice of complex paediatric cardiac surgery at the Bristol Royal Infirmary between 1990 and 1995, although concerns went back to 1984. As the independent inquiry, published later in July 2001, said in its opening summary:[1]

> The story of the paediatric cardiac surgical service in Bristol is not an account of bad people. Nor is it an account of people who did not care, nor of people who wilfully harm patients. It is an account of people

who cared greatly about human suffering, and were dedicated and were well motivated. Sadly, some lacked insight and their behaviour was flawed. Many failed to communicate with each other, and to work together effectively for the interests of their patients. There was lack of leadership, and of teamwork.

The inquiry placed the issues in their wider context, describing 'health-care professionals working in Bristol who were victims of a combination of circumstances that owed as much to general failings in the NHS at the time than to any individual failing. Despite their manifest good intentions and long hours of dedicated work, there were failures on occasion in the care provided to very sick children.'

The events at Bristol, as revealed through the evidence at the GMC hearing, triggered huge changes not only in the regulation of doctors, but in the organisation, governance and capacity of the National Health Service (NHS). It provoked in a major way the further development of a new professionalism for medicine. In a leader[2] in the *British Medical Journal* (*BMJ*) at the conclusion of the hearing, the Editor Richard Smith quoted Yeats' memorable words, 'All changed, changed utterly.' And so it was to be.

Part 1
What, why,
who and how

1

Introduction

This book is about the changing relationship between the public and their doctors. Most of us at one time or another, either directly or through others, have appreciated the benefits of modern medicine. Moreover, right up to the present day, survey after survey has shown that doctors as an occupational group are regarded as more trustworthy than most others, indicating that many patients have good personal relationships with those who treat them. That undoubtedly reflects the fact that most doctors are still strongly vocationally motivated to do the best for their patients. Their pressing priority is getting the conditions right for effective practice. In an NHS seriously short of doctors, time is at a premium. Most doctors want to have time to talk to their patients properly, to empathise, to listen, to explain, to reassure and to help put people at ease in what are often frightening situations. They want to practise in modern, well-equipped facilities. They want to be proud of their professionalism with all that it stands for in terms of assuring quality and being properly accountable.

And yet clearly something has gone wrong. Bristol and several other major cases of poor or bad performance came to light in the 1990s over a short period of time and with huge publicity. They raised serious questions in the public mind both about the individual doctors concerned and also about the culture and practices of medicine and institutional management in the NHS and the private sector. In particular the medical profession's own arrangements for regulating its members, and the Government's structure and systems for assuring patient safety and quality in the NHS and the private sector, were shown to be inadequate. So much of the health service seemed to work well more as a result of the conscientiousness of individual clinicians than of the design and reliability of the professional and management systems for ensuring quality and safety – and the public could sense that. Perhaps this explains how the public at large can speak critically of the medical profession whilst patients are positive about 'their' doctor.

So how did this situation come about? Public confidence in a profession is sustained when its expectations are – or are perceived to be – in harmony with professional culture and actual performance. On the other hand, public confidence is undermined when a significant gap appears between general expectation and performance. This is what happened to the medical profession in the later years of the 20th century. Essentially it remained wedded to a 19th century concept of a professional culture at a time when society had moved on. Even though throughout the whole of the 20th century the profession was vigorously progressive in developing medical science and technology, it remained collectively deeply conservative in matters of attitude and human relationships. For example, it continued to see itself as the dominant partner in the doctor/patient/public relationship and in the organisation of medical work, even though the need for teamworking had been recognised for some time. The notion of unrestricted clinical autonomy, previously unquestioned by most patients as well as doctors, still lingered despite the emergence of evidence-based medicine and new societal expectations of professional accountability. So the medical profession missed the point – and it was certainly not the only one to do so – that paternalism, even where it was benign, was becoming less acceptable in a consumer society in which patient/customer/client autonomy was emerging as the new order. Hence the growing criticism of a profession that was seen to be introspective, to be limited in its willingness and ability to communicate effectively, secretive about risks and variations in performance, and unwilling to admit to – and where necessary apologise for – the errors which are inherent in judgement-based clinical decision making.

Nowhere is this changing relationship illustrated better than in medical and societal attitudes to consent. In an era when patients deferred to doctors – and this was most of the last century – doctors often assumed consent. In such a climate organs could be removed (for sound reasons), or organs and tissue could be kept for teaching and research – all without asking patients. But society moved on. For the public consent became a statement about the doctor–patient relationship, a touchstone signalling respect for the autonomy of the patient in all its dimensions as well as permission for a particular procedure. For those doctors who did not see or recognise the change, medicine was 'not what it used to be' and they labelled patients who asserted their right to appropriate behaviours from doctors as 'awkward' or 'demanding.'

Although professional culture was the starting point, it did not itself account fully for the problem of medical failures. Other factors were impinging on a profession and healthcare system that was already trying to adapt to the modern world. Indeed it is now clear that there was an overall systems failure in healthcare generally. Complacent institutional governance, the lack of independent external institutional regulation and an amazing lack of useable data on performance at all levels of healthcare provision in the NHS and indeed the private sector, were symptomatic and contributed significantly. So systems matter. But it is people, individually and collectively, who design systems and operate them. It is people who are in charge of them. We are therefore always driven back ultimately to culture and human behaviour, not just of doctors, but also of managers, politicians, other health professionals and patients themselves.

In 1994 the Chief Medical Officer for England, Sir Kenneth Calman, urged the medical profession to look beyond its present depressed circumstances to the future. He, like myself, believed that the profession had to modernise its ideas about its professionalism.[3] The result of his urging was a 'summit' meeting that year of the profession, the first since 1961, to consider medicine's core values. At that conference Sir Maurice Shock,[4] former rector of Lincoln College, Oxford, said that doctors seemed to imagine that they were living in Gladstone's world of minimal government, benign self-regulation and a self-effacing state. They had been completely unprepared for the consumerist 'blitzkrieg from the right' that had overwhelmed them at the end of the 1980s. I was present and for me what was striking about that conference was that it was the profession talking to itself. The participants were mainly middle-aged men. I do not remember any doctors from ethnic minorities. Patient representatives were few and far between. In a way this seemed merely to exemplify the cultural gap.

It is against this background that Bristol and all that lay behind it came to be seen as such a major watershed in the relationship between the medical profession and the public. Sadly, it seems that it takes disasters like Bristol to bring about or speed up change. We see it in so many other walks of life. It took the *Herald of Free Enterprise* disaster to shake up safety regulations in the shipping world, the Guinness scandal, Enron and Worldcom to stimulate reform in financial services, the Chernobyl catastrophe to awaken the world to nuclear safety. So it was with the medical profession and the NHS where a producer-dominated culture needed a strong jolt to overcome resistance to the new realities of life.

However, it is helpful to remember that the adjustments required of the medical profession in this country had their parallels elsewhere in the world. We were not unique, as those who live in Canada, the USA, Australia, Germany, and France and elsewhere all know. What was really happening was a worldwide change in the relationship between the public and doctors as traditional paternalism in all its guises began to be displaced by patient-centred care.*

* This is not peculiar to the Western world or societies where the public is articulate and assertive. In a British Council workshop held in September 2002, my wife Sally and I, who were joint directors of the event, discovered that doctors and administrators from countries like Egypt, Malaysia, China, Taiwan, Nigeria, Ghana, Korea, Grenada and Myanmar were all looking to refocus their healthcare on patient needs and wants rather than doctors', irrespective of whether the population was demanding it or not.

This book

I start from a very simple premise. When we are ill we want to know that we have a good doctor whose technical knowledge and skills we can be sure of, on whose honesty we can rely, and who will treat us empathetically with the respect and courtesy to which we are entitled. We need to be sure that the hospital or primary care team to which our doctor usually belongs works effectively and safely so we can be assured that we are getting care of good quality. And we need good access to care. My story is primarily about the first of the two – doctors' professionalism, and good governance in clinical teams. Access is more about the capacity of the system, and is therefore beyond my scope. In this book I ask what further changes have to be made to the culture and regulation of the medical profession to make it as trustworthy as the public would like, and indeed are entitled to expect. The book focuses on the GMC because it was a mirror of the culture of a self-regulated profession, and therefore illustrates how that change process has been developed and pursued.

Two things prompted me to write the book. First I wanted to tell the story of the changing relationship between doctors and the public as I have witnessed and experienced it. In particular, I wanted to describe the reasons why and how professional regulation, both through the GMC and doctors' NHS contracts, failed to protect patients adequately from poorly performing doctors, and what lessons we can learn from that. In a sense it is my personal testimony, my own observation, analysis and interpretation of a particular period in medicine in the UK. The story reaches back beyond my 38 years as a practising doctor. But the book relates primarily to the period in the late 1990s when matters reached a climax. As President of the GMC between 1995 and 2002, I had an unrivalled view of the action 'from the bridge' and, indeed, was a significant contributor to some of the events.

I have attempted to describe the main issues and happenings. Inevitably the account is partial, and no doubt there will be others who will contribute their perspective to an important time in the history of the medical profession. Some of the processes I describe in these pages were emotionally bloody because the inbuilt inertia was formidable. But in that frenetic period the new ethos of professional regulation that emerged put the interests of patients firmly at the heart of things. It embodied a new approach to medical professionalism, founded on a partnership between the public and doctors.

The struggle to achieve agreement about the new public–profession relationship was brought to a head in the aftermath of Bristol over the GMC's proposal for revalidation. This requirement, that affected every doctor, involved a major change in the medical culture. Until that time a doctor's registration with the GMC was based on historical evidence –

gathered often many years earlier – on first joining the Medical Register. In future, the GMC said doctors would have to provide evidence regularly that they remained up to date and fit to practise if they wanted to keep their registration, that is, their licence to practice. They would have to 'revalidate' that registration. Many amongst the public thought that happened anyway, and were surprised that it did not. In the event some doctors objected on principle. Within the much bigger group that accepted the principle there were shades of opinion about how robust the process should be. The minimalists who still hankered after the old style of medicine wanted to do the least possible consistent with good appearances – they saw revalidation as an unwelcome imposition. The maximalists wanted to be open and rigorous in furnishing the evidence about their practice, seeing this as an expression of respect for their patients and themselves in tune with the public's ideas of professional accountability. As a general practitioner and lately as President of the GMC, I was part of the struggle – a maximalist throughout.

That brings me to the second reason for this book. As it is published, the reconstituted and reconstructed regulator of the profession, the new GMC, is coming into action. That is good news. Nevertheless there is more work to be done before this cultural revolution is over, and in the last chapter I raise some of the still outstanding issues and what could be done about them.

This book has been written for anyone – member of the public or doctor – who is interested in what may be seen as an important moment in the history of medicine in the UK. I try to give the reader an insight into the medical profession, its culture and what makes it tick. Because I believe that culture is so central, the book is primarily about the medical tribe, what it is, its institutions, and highlights its strengths and those characteristics that sowed the seeds of future trouble. In particular I wanted to convey how it felt going through that process of achieving change whilst it was still fresh in my mind and as a member of a proud profession that was feeling shell-shocked, confused and resentful towards an NHS that seemed incapable of creating the working conditions and environment in which 'proper doctoring' could flourish.

As a testimony it is inevitably a mixture of monograph and bio-graphical style. I felt it was essential to provide an outline of the historical context, without which the later events would not make much sense, particularly to readers who are not familiar with it. Those who know the context must forgive me. It becomes more biographical in style as we reach the recent events where I had a particular knowledge and perspect-ive, seen through the lens of my own experience, first as a general practitioner and finally as the President of the GMC.

I have been involved throughout most of my professional life in trying to bring about this change in culture. Securing the new culture is fundamental to re-establishing public confidence, not only in doctors but also in the healthcare system. Better regulation, better systems, proper investment and adequate capacity will all help, but of themselves will not achieve optimum results for the public. Doctors, individually and collectively, need to equate professionalism with quality in healthcare, to feel passionately about them both, to take ownership of the ideas, systems and methods, and make them work well. They need to do this in a new partnership with the public and with the health professionals and managers with whom they work. There lies the way forward.

2

Life in medicine

In 1995, I stood for election as President of the GMC on a programme of reform both of professionalism in medicine and the GMC itself. There were members within the GMC, both medical and lay, who believed that such reform of the GMC had to be carried out swiftly. Otherwise public confidence in the medical profession, and in particular in the system of professional self-regulation, for which the GMC was primarily responsible, could not be sustained. As it stood, the system, notwithstanding some important new developments, was riding for a fall.

In the early 1990s there were already signs of a new vision of medical professionalism, regulation and quality in healthcare emerging in the UK, what the medical sociologist Margaret Stacey called a 'new professionalism' in medicine.[5] I was very much part of that new vision.[6,7] For me it would be critical when the going got rough in order to sustain my sense of purpose and direction. It would strengthen my determination to carry through a radical reform agenda despite the turbulence within the profession that would create. In making cultural change some clashes are inevitable.

This chapter is a brief account of the key influences in my professional life that shaped my thinking. It shows the significant bearing they had on how I saw my profession and its responsibilities to society, both when I took office as the GMC's President and in my subsequent analysis and handling of the situation as it unfolded.

Early experience

The earliest influence was from being a patient. As a ten-year-old child I had had experience of being ill. I developed rheumatic fever, which was then a serious illness because of the possible heart complications. I was in bed for six months and absent from school for a year. I remember vividly the start of pericarditis* – 'a marble in my chest' was how I described it. We were on holiday in Edinburgh. The paediatrician who was called in

* The inflammation of the sac around the heart.

was the late Charles McNeil, Professor of Child Health at Edinburgh University. I remember him as a very kind man who made me feel both that I was special and that I would get better. His technical abilities meant nothing to me as a child – he was simply the doctor. I was to see that experience mirrored throughout my professional life in patients who accepted technical competence as given, and made the judgement of a doctor on the quality of the relationship they established.

I grew up in a medical household. My father was a general practitioner in the coal-mining community of Ashington in Northumberland. Everyone, myself included, expected me to become a doctor. Family succession was still common in those days. So I qualified in medicine at the University of Durham in Newcastle upon Tyne* in 1958 with the intention of joining him.

Medical teaching was very much in the hands of the consultants who were on the staff of the teaching hospital – the Royal Victoria Infirmary – and its associated hospitals. Unusually, Newcastle had a department of child health with strong community leanings, so we were exposed to the importance of the social dimension of illness in children. It is often said that medical teaching by humiliation was prevalent in that era. I witnessed that only rarely. The vast majority of registrars and consultants who did the teaching were quite dedicated and I saw many acts of kindness to patients. There was, however, a powerful aura of élitism. Consultants working at the teaching hospital regarded themselves as the élite of medicine.

Consultants in district hospitals,† and below them the doctors in public health medicine and general practice, were in a clear pecking order. If you wanted to get to 'the top' in medicine you had to become a consultant at a teaching hospital. Moreover, a teaching hospital appointment was crucial to private practice. Doctors were prepared to hold themselves back for years in senior registrar posts waiting for the right job to become vacant. At that time the teaching hospital consultants had little understanding of patients' lives outside hospital and therefore had a seriously limited knowledge of the nature of the clinical work in general practice and, to an extent, in public health medicine. Yet the basic medical school training of a doctor was designed to produce a safe general practitioner. Further training followed only for those who were going to specialise.

A very personal practice

After two years of hospital experience I joined my father as a principal in general practice in 1960. My father had bought the goodwill of the

---

* Shortly to become the Medical School in the University of Newcastle upon Tyne.
† There were not so many then as there are now.

practice in 1931. He was single-handed, as most general practitioners were at that time. In the inter-war years, coal mining was seriously depressed. It was tough, demanding and dangerous work for the miners and it was hard on the women who sustained their men and brought up the children. Those severe economic conditions had eased somewhat by the time I joined the practice – coal mining had become a better-paid job. Nevertheless, morbidity in that community was high and there were pockets of some of the most deprived people in the country.

As a community, Ashington was very close-knit. Like most of the mining villages of the north east of England, it was relatively closed with inter-connecting families and therefore a network of personal relationships. As a doctor in that kind of community you soon learnt the value of the networks of patient care, especially of children, the elderly and people with chronic illness and handicap. You also very soon learnt the practical necessity of confidentiality – for your words would be fed into the network and you could never be sure where injudicious remarks about people and their illnesses might end up!

My father and I practised together for nine years before he retired through ill health. He was deeply respected by his patients – a respect built up over the years and founded on confidence in his diagnosis and treatment, and especially an enviable reputation for unstinting service to people, through thick and thin, when they were ill. He did not walk away when medical treatment had nothing more to offer. He knew the limits of his knowledge and skill as a doctor and practised strictly within them. He built up a relationship with most of the consultants to whom he referred patients (there were fewer consultants then) and he taught me the niceties of deciding which consultant to recommend to patients and of protecting patients from the overzealous specialist. He was a true family doctor and a hard act to follow. Even as I retired from the practice nearly 30 years later, people of the older generation still remembered him as 'the doctor'.

My father had a system of daily patient review, the like of which I have never seen elsewhere. In those days many very sick people were looked after by relatives in their own homes. A daily visiting list would include about 20 house calls for each doctor. My father kept a large monthly visiting ledger, showing which of us had seen which patient and when the next visit was due. At the end of each consulting day – around 7 p.m. – for the next hour or so we would 'make up the list' of patients seen at home. We exchanged information about each patient, and tricky clinical problems were talked over. We would regularly see each other's patients, mainly to ensure we both knew all the patients who were seriously ill, but also, if we had doubts, to have a quick second opinion. My father regarded this as a normal part of the clinical process – all about 'knowing your practice', 'knowing your patients' and being 'on top of the job'. It was another pair of eyes in what was otherwise a single-handed practice. Today we would call it part of good practice-based clinical governance.

It was in those early years that I had to confront, personally, some of the then dominant features of the medical culture in which I had been brought up by the medical specialists who had taught me. For example, the received wisdom was that patients with terminal illness should not be told. Exceptions were businessmen who for some strange reason were thought to be the only people who needed to put their affairs in order. That approach had seemed fine in hospital. But I found it increasingly difficult to visit dying patients in their homes and, in the intimacy of that setting, collude with the family against the patient. Too often I felt that patients I looked after knew or suspected the truth, but neither of us would say. In the end I had to break free from this cultural straight-jacket. I found that establishing a relationship based on honesty was far better for all concerned.* It removed a barrier which, I learnt, had too often prevented real conversation between the patient and their closest loved ones. I learnt too that the more experience I gained of handling patients with serious illness, particularly cancer for which treatment was very limited, the more difficult it actually was to predict how people would react to bad news. I was as often as not wrong in my predictions.

The result was that patients had more responsibility and freedom in deciding on their care. This was beautifully illustrated when an elderly patient of mine developed cancer of the lung. We talked about the treatment options and he chose to do nothing. He would take his chance. Five years later – still alive and with a good quality of life – he had a bladder complaint investigated. The surgeon was surprised that he had had no treatment for his lung cancer. 'You fix my bladder,' said the patient to the surgeon, 'and leave my cancer to me and my maker.' Later, near to death from the cancer, he said to me, 'Donald, I made the right decision.' The surgeon did not understand how a patient could opt in such circumstances to take no action. Who can say who was right? It was this kind of experience which convinced me that my medical training had not equipped me properly for the job. It led directly to my involvement in the new vocational training for general practice, the ideas for which were beginning to be shaped by some more senior general practitioners who felt similarly.

In that close-knit community, relationships and performance as a doctor mattered. Health, illness and what the doctor had said or done – or had not said or done – were main staples of conversation at the surgery, in the shops, at the working men's clubs, on the bus and so on. In everyday life there was an endless swapping of stories, anecdotes and gossip about people's experiences. Through this, patients and their

---

* That sounds obvious and easy, but it was not. The cultural mores were very strong.

families adjudicated on your standards and reputation as a doctor. It is often said that patients cannot judge a doctor clinically. But that, in my experience, is only partially true. People in Ashington may not indeed have understood the technicalities, but they could certainly judge the process. Was young Annie's meningitis picked up early enough? Did the doctor respond promptly to Uncle Joe's chest pain? People had their own ideas about whether they had had 'a good examination'. And everybody, all but the very young, had an opinion on the doctor's manner. So the patient's perspective on these things was not just interesting, it was important. Through direct experience it gave their view of a doctor's performance. Every doctor in our town was categorised. Comparisons, at times pointed and uncomfortable for the recipients, were made, and came back not infrequently via others. And that information was fed to newcomers who would enquire of their neighbours who was the best doctor. Listening to 'the word on the street' was how people normally chose a doctor. It is the method that most doctors I know use today when choosing a colleague to attend their families or themselves.

These kinds of experiences confirmed in my mind just how important is the patient's assessment of the doctor's performance and therefore how essential it is that patients have choice. People need to have doctors that they feel they can trust technically and that they feel comfortable with. Empathy matters. Being respected matters. Personality matters, especially in the management of chronic illness where longer-term relationships are usually involved.

Lintonville Medical Group

In 1969 my father retired and I joined forces with colleagues in two other small practices. By this time I was fully involved in the arrangements being made in general practice for the new vocational training. We established Lintonville as a multidisciplinary teaching practice – a new idea then. My partners and I committed ourselves explicitly from the outset to try to provide a good standard of primary care. To this end we signed up to the principles of standard setting and performance monitoring which other general practitioner teachers and I were establishing as the norm for the new training practices. The teachers set these standards of the day through the College of General Practitioners (later the RCGP) and implemented them through the new university postgraduate training organisations that we were establishing for general practice. So as a practice, we became regularly involved in internal and external medical and multidisciplinary audit, which were also new. It meant accepting a regular external review of practice standards by our peers, to try to answer the question 'Do we practise what we teach?'

In the 1980s the rising workload in general practice was a serious problem. It had consequences for patient access and our quality of professional life. 'Finger in the dyke' measures had proved useless. We had to find better ways of managing all our resources – people, time, energy, finances, data. We learnt the hard way the value of setting clear operating standards and of having performance data which would enable us to diagnose operational problems properly, set the levels of performance to which we aspired and tell us whether we were achieving them. This way we learnt the value of audit as a management tool. The insights revealed by the data and the discipline of operating standards forced us to think about new working patterns and new forms of teamworking to achieve our objective.

In the 1980s Sally Fountain (now Irvine), then General Administrator of the RCGP, and June Huntington of the King's Fund began to work closely together. They were to bring to primary care insights as to how general management principles could enhance teamworking and, ultimately, the delivery and indeed the quality of clinical care and outcome. In 1989, having had the benefit of Sally's advice directly, our practice underwent a major reorganisation to embody, as far as we felt able, modern management practices. We learnt from that just how important good management was, particularly to planned preventive care and the care of patients with chronic illness. It helped us to 'know our practice', to be 'on top of the job', as my father put it. We began to see management much more clearly not as something others did to us, but as an integral and indispensable part of our professionalism.

In the early 1990s we became 'fundholders.' We thought it was a great idea. It was one of the most innovative of the Conservative Government's NHS reforms, designed to put patients first through an internal market. In this scheme we assumed responsibility for the purchase of secondary care for our patients. We became responsible for our prescribing and practice team budgets. But we were interested primarily in the opportunity fundholding created to develop our primary care. As a practice we saw ourselves ultimately as contractors delivering a given range, volume and quality of primary care against an agreed price and the purchase of secondary hospital care on behalf of our patients.* Fundholding brought new investment into the practice, to strengthen the infrastructure so that managing for quality improvement came a step closer to operational

---

* Later that became possible. Nowadays, practices like Lintonville working within Personal Medical Services (PMS) pilots, an evolutionary development of fundholding, are similarly responsible for delivering a contract from the health authority for all personal medical services for the practice population. PMS practices are judged by their performance but have substantial discretion about how they organise themselves to deliver the contract. This creates major opportunities for experimentation and individual practice innovation and new thinking.

reality. We strengthened our data sources through a second-generation practice computer system. The result was better clinical management, more informed by data that started to become available on our performance as a practice. Clinical audit became fully embedded in the practice as a management as well as a learning tool, yielding practical, year by year improvements in, for instance, the care of patients with diabetes, and raised blood pressure, and in our practice of preventive medicine. We tested ourselves as a group and individually against external markers such as the quality standard *ISO 9002* and *Fellowship by Assessment* of the RCGP. Above all the whole team participated both in achieving and in celebrating its success.

We took a big step forward on teamworking. By now there were five partners, two associates and two trainee general practitioners. But the whole team consisted of over 50 people. So attention to teamworking was vital. We invested heavily in time and effort to get practical teamworking as effective as possible for patients. There were new developments. For example, we trained a health visitor to become a full nurse practitioner and we established a professional development fund, open to all members of the practice team, from savings generated by fundholding. This was to help any team member develop knowledge and skills that would improve the patient services of the practice. It was a good motivator, especially for practice staff for whose professional development the NHS had provided most inadequately. It gave a return, in terms of morale as well as professional development, out of all proportion to the quite modest sums involved.

The fundholding era saw our first foray into patient surveys. Working with the forward-looking Northumberland Family Practitioner Committee (FPC), we surveyed a representative sample of the practice population to find out what patients thought about our services. The results were at once reassuring and uncomfortable. They were reassuring about the patients' perception of the quality of clinical care but showed what we needed to do better, particularly about access – for example, wheelchair access was a problem. It taught us the value of asking patients directly about their experience and it led to improvements we would not otherwise have made.

One of the important innovations in 1989, highly germane to this book, was the decision to give everyone in the team permission to raise sensitive questions about critical incidents that worried them. We established a simple mechanism for handling these in a 'no-blame' environment that would lead to prompt internal inquiry, investigation and action. At that time we saw this as an important part of making clinical care as safe and acceptable as possible, of minimising our exposure to clinical risk and where necessary making improvements.

We were a happy practice. We saw our quality-improving activities as an asset, despite a heavy clinical workload. They helped us to see how well we were doing and where improvement was needed, which strengthened our sense of professionalism and our feelings of self-respect. Ownership was a strong motivator. For us good leadership, a strong patient-oriented outlook, health professionals who were good at their jobs, good teamworking, management and audit were all essential ingredients of high morale. But so was the freedom to organise and manage our own work as a practice around our patients' needs, not around government targets. Today, seen from a now very wide experience of general practice, those very characteristics seem to mark out happy practices that are largely 'on top of the job', 'know their patients' and retain substantial control of their work from the unhappy ones which are driven by outside forces.

My practice experience was fundamental to my thinking on professionalism, quality care and the interface with management. It was this experience, more than any other, which revealed to me and convinced me of the vital importance of integrating management with clinical standard setting and internal quality assurance. It was good for the morale of the clinical team and good for patients. Furthermore, the more a clinical team could demonstrate individual and collective performance as a normal part of its business, the less necessity or justification there was for heavy, intrusive external review. This would be highly relevant when I came later to deal with the thorny questions around clinical governance and the evidence required for the revalidation of doctors' registration.

The care of patients remained my core function throughout my professional life, until I retired from active practice to become GMC President. Clinical practice was the part of medicine that I enjoyed most. It was the real world.

The impact of vocational training

The kinds of practice developments that occurred at Lintonville did not happen in isolation. I was one of the founders of the new vocational training for general practice, and through this I contributed to bringing a new kind of professionalism to medical education in this country. I was involved at three levels: teaching in the practice, the provision and organisation of training with Newcastle University and nationally with the RCGP.

Vocational training, though never designed as such, soon became a test bed and a vehicle for trying out new ideas about general practice. The regions were the places where these ideas were applied in practice. As a Regional Advisor in General Practice* I worked with some wonderful

---

* Now these posts as known as part of the NHS civil service, and are renamed Directors of Postgraduate General Practice Education.

colleagues. We began in 1969 with six practices.* There were eventually 68 teaching practices involved in vocational training in the Northern Region.

Across the country, especially in those early days, there was strong informal competition between the regions, and schemes within the regions that drove up standards. We took pride in our national – and later international – reputation.

One of the most important consequences of vocational training was the introduction, from the very beginning, of a system of standard setting and external performance review in the teaching practices. We were determined that trainees would be placed only in practices that were known to provide a good standard of patient care, and that would take teaching seriously. In the 25 years that I was involved in the programme, I learnt how it was possible to secure peer agreement to high professional standards for trainers and their practices, and to run a tight, peer-driven system of professional regulation.

Leadership was fundamental to sustaining and developing that professional culture. Trainers were selected partly for their leadership qualities in their practices. They were important role models. Leadership mattered in those who helped to run training schemes. A great deal of effort went into the professional development of the teaching workforce through informal trainers networks, regular workshops, clinical standard setting, and audit activities and so on. We saw serious investment of time, effort and money in the professional development of the teachers and their practices as fundamental. I regarded them as 'the gold in the bank', the key to successful vocational training.

Let me give just one example. In 1974 we started one of the first clinical audit groups in the country. Our aim was to sensitise ourselves to the review of our clinical work in peer groups, to try to learn how to accept criticisms without being hurt, to give it without offence and to change our practice behaviour where necessary. We looked at our own cases where diagnosis and management might have been better, randomly chosen clinical records for their quality, an elementary audit of the treatment of urinary tract infection and, on occasions, the presentation of cases where the doctor knew things had gone wrong. The people taking part (ultimately and for a while there were about a hundred) were very enthusiastic. It was this kind of experience that was crucial to cultural development, although we did not think of it in those terms then.

So this taught me one of the most important lessons of my career. Setting clear professional standards, by agreement with those concerned, was a valuable – and valued – activity. People knew what was expected

---

* Training was started originally by Andrew Smith, Aubrey Colling, John Walker, Michael McKendrick and myself in two centres, one in Northumberland and one in Stockton.

of them. They signed up. In addition there had to be a regulatory framework that involved regular monitoring and review – are we doing what we promised? But it could not be left there. Crucially between these two bookends, it was the sustained effort through small, well-led groups to help trainers help themselves to keep moving forward, to develop and hone their professionalism, that really mattered. It made the difference between minimalism and maximalism, doing the least the rules require and giving unstintingly of one's best.

Disseminating ideas

I set out these ideas in a series of papers and books starting in 1975, when I first proposed that there had to be action to deal with the large tail of poorly performing doctors in general practice. I proposed the RCGP *Quality Initiative* in 1982, which became a serious attempt by the College, led by its council, to confront the problem of poor practice by promoting and demonstrating good practice. The route was through the positive act of establishing standard setting and performance monitoring as professionally the right thing to do for all in general practice, just as I have described earlier. In the late 1980s I chaired the first national study of standard setting and performance monitoring in general practice, in the teaching practices in the Northern Region, and during the 1990s I published a series of papers and books developing my ideas and experiences of quality and professionalism in medical practice.

Wider influences

We are all the creatures of our experiences and I was influenced constantly over the years by what patients told me they thought about their care, in my own practice and much more generally when I was President of the GMC.

The biggest influence by far was other doctors, many of whom occur in this story. The most sustained influences came from my medical and non-medical colleagues in my practice, my fellow-teachers in the Northern Region and my colleagues at the RCGP. What we did we did together – it was very much a team enterprise.

The social scientists, collectively, were an important influence. The late Professor Margot Jeffreys, the first medical sociologist in the UK, taught me in my younger days through our many conversations about the value of the sociological perspective on the behaviour of doctors and of the kind of sociological methods that could be used to study that. On quality assessment, Avedis Donabedian, the doyen and champion of patient-oriented quality in the USA, was deeply influential. Through him I became an avid student of the literature and practice on quality assessment and on professionalism. In Newcastle, Ian Russell, a medical statistician and health services researcher, was a tremendously influential working colleague who introduced me to the new technologies of clinical guideline construction and clinical performance assessment. The writings of the American sociologist Eliot Freidson were I thought seminal, particularly on his insights into the medical culture. The studies of another American sociologist, Marilynn Rosenthal, on dysfunctional doctors and on the dysfunctional arrangements for handling complaints against doctors in the NHS in the early 1990s laid out the problem more clearly than any other, and were thus strongly influential. Rudolph Klein always provided food for thought in his writings on standards in healthcare, and has given me good advice over the years. And I have mentioned Margaret Stacey already. Her refreshing, scholarly yet stimulating approach to the reform of medical regulation through the GMC I greatly admired.

So this was my world, in which I developed my own ideas about the future development of the medical profession.

3

The medical tribe

I am one of some 200 000 doctors on the GMC register, about half of whom are practising in this country, mainly in the NHS. The remainder are either retired, working outside medicine or live overseas. Roughly a third of the UK practising doctors are general practitioners, a third are consultants in the hospital specialities and public health medicine and a third are in training or support posts.

Most doctors have a shared understanding of what being a doctor is all about. Medicine is first and foremost a clinical profession. Doctors exist primarily to diagnose patients' problems and where possible treat them – all else is subsidiary. Diagnosis separates doctors from the other health professionals. Doctors are clinical problem solvers, trained to unravel a set of symptoms and physical signs into coherent recognisable patterns of disease.

Because of the complexity of medicine, diagnosis is seriously challenging and demanding, and it can be nerve-wracking. Doctors, unlike for example theoretical scientists, do not have the opportunity to collect evidence and draw conclusions in a measured and comprehensive way, even though a high value is placed on scientific knowledge. On the contrary, because of the nature of people and the way that illness presents, doctors often have to make decisions – even if it is a decision to do nothing – on clinical data that are normally incomplete. Like most doctors, I have worried whether the child who has a headache is in fact suffering from the onset of a minor infection or meningitis. Is the vague pain in that man's chest a symptom of heart disease or indigestion? This kind of problem solving involves considerable judgement and pragmatism as the process of unravelling the problem follows its course often over some time. It is therefore prone to error.

Clinical decision making is still very personal. Hence the core beliefs of 'clinical autonomy' and 'clinical freedom' that derive from the doctor's duty to make diagnostic and treatment decisions that are deemed by the individual doctor to be in the patient's best interest. An important issue today is how far clinical autonomy should be restrained within the boundaries of evidence-based medicine, whilst leaving the doctor sufficient discretion to get it right for individuals whose response to disease may subtly differ from one patient to another.

Clinical uncertainty, combined with the fact that doctors generally still make most clinical decisions on their own, is at the root of many of the defensive reactions to error. Clinical pragmatism, and the need to retain the confidence of the patient and the doctor's need to feel confident themselves, are the seeds of ultimate rationalisation if things go wrong subsequently. If the doctor is not prepared to confront and deal with an error when it happens, it can be the starting point of personal denial of the truth. Rationalisation expressed as 'I couldn't help it' and 'there were unexpected circumstances' are common reactions. Denial is also the starting point of collusive behaviour – 'there but for the grace of God, go I.'

Having said that, clinical decision making in skilled hands is almost an art form.

Tribal characteristics

The modern medical profession is built around the unifying theme of a common pathway to becoming a doctor in the UK. That intensive five-year apprenticeship and academic course is where medical students absorb the culture of the medical profession from their teachers. It is in that period that the intense process of medicalisation begins. It is at once a strength and a weakness. It is a strength in that it reinforces the cultural attitudes and practices that by common consent are deemed good for patients. It is a weakness in that it can reinforce behaviours and attitudes that students observe in teachers, which are either not in harmony with patient expectations or at variance with safe practice. In medical training especially, role modelling is a powerful influence, for better or worse.

Since World War II, of doctors registered for the first time each year, about half have been trained outside the UK. Of doctors working in the NHS, about 25% have been trained outside the UK. Pragmatically, the assumption has been made that graduates from other countries with widely differing cultural backgrounds would have or would assume the characteristics of the indigenous tribe. This could never be so.

There have been some unhelpful characteristics in the medical profession that are relevant to this story. They include:

- a strong general culture of self-protection, defending the group and individual transgressors against outside criticism or attack except where deviant behaviour has been explicitly acknowledged by the tribe as unacceptable. Examples of such tribal behaviour by individuals against the majority have included unreasonable advertising, denigrating a colleague's practice and 'poaching' a colleague's patients, that is to say any behaviours that impinge on a colleague's livelihood. These varied examples come under the heading of protecting livelihoods and reputations.

- a particular culture of élitism, founded on high performance as a diagnostician/technician/scientist, which by a process of self and group selection came to dominate the medical schools, especially in the early years of the NHS. This culture, to which all students were exposed, had obvious strengths but was dismissive of failure. Sir Lancelot Spratt, the grand surgeon in the book and film *Doctor in the House*,* was the caricature based on reality.
- of particular relevance to this book is the misplaced collegiality which results in the tendency to defend the clinical practice of individual members except in the most flagrant circumstances. 'There but for the grace of God, go I', to which I referred earlier, may be coupled with the simpler 'not my problem'. Both are prescriptions for inaction.
- the complex behaviour of a profession whose outward reputation is dependent primarily on the exercise of skill, judgement and diagnostic accuracy and therefore being right, yet has to handle the serious stresses and strains imposed on individuals who may feel torn between preserving their reputation and revealing their own feelings of fallibility or uncertainty.
- consequent on this, a professional culture in which the admission of error has been seen as difficult, the act of apologising as defensive and weak, and the entitlement of people to know about the circumstances of error not readily conceded.
- within the last 30 years in particular, because of a wholly understandable focus on the new science and its obvious benefits for patients, a relative lack of attention to personal attitudes and conduct, particularly to matters of consent and communication with patients and their relatives, which simply fuels the perception of a doctor as paternalistic, detached or arrogant.†

Most doctors find these issues very sensitive and difficult to handle. Medical training has been weak on how to deal with, for example,

---

* By Richard Gordon, later filmed with James Robertson Justice as Lancelot Spratt.

† In 1975, an anxious consultant at a meeting took me aside privately to ask whether a video of him consulting could be arranged as he wanted to know how he behaved with patients. We made much use of videoed consultations at the time in general practice. I arranged it, but asked him why the private conversation. He said, 'I dare not raise it with my [consultant] colleagues. They would think me soft.' I learnt about the intimidating power of the culture from that incident.

unfavourable or bad outcomes for a patient, or criticisms made by anybody. Indeed, a central part of my discussions with medical schools in my presidency at the GMC was how to get to grips with the reality of these challenging cultural characteristics. Finding ways of modifying their impact, or in some circumstances removing them, is part of the story of this book.

Tribal origins

Now I want to step back, to look a little more clearly at the origins of the modern medical profession in the UK, and some of the tribal behaviour that contributes to its culture. This is not intended as a history of medicine but some facts help to explain the context. I have drawn particularly on the work of Rosemary Stevens,[8] whose wonderful book on the development of medical practice in England I have dipped into regularly throughout my professional life.

It may seem very surprising in the light of the prominent position of doctors in society today that actually the modern medical profession is relatively young – around 150 or so years of age. Until the mid-18th century quacks performed with leeches, quasi-scientists examined George III's stools and barber surgeons pulled teeth and cut off limbs. But the medical profession as we would recognise it began to evolve quickly in the second half of the 19th century on the back of scientific and technological discovery – for example Lister and antisepsis, Koch and the identification of tuberculosis. It was during this time that the great diagnostic clinicians began to emerge, meticulously describing and documenting the pictures of illness – Sydenham, Huntington, Parkinson and many others. Medicine at its leading edge was beginning to take shape as a 'profession', at the heart of which was a growing body of scientific knowledge about the structure and functions of the human body and of disease, the mastery of which required special qualities and skills.

In the mid 19th century the practice of medicine had developed to a point where it was beginning to be seen as a boon and a major contributor to the health and well-being of society. One major consequence was that the newly found professional status of doctors was given special recognition by Parliament in the form of the Medical Act of 1858. That Act unified the various disparate groups of doctors into a single profession. It formalised the power of the profession through the new General Medical Council to decide who could be in that profession and who could not.

Prior to the Act the medical profession had been evolving over the years along two main tracks. There were physicians and surgeons who were the forerunners of today's hospital consultants, and there were the apothecaries who were the predecessors of today's general practitioners.

These groups had different social origins. For example, members of the Royal College of Physicians of London (RCP) were drawn from the upper strata of society, and ministered only to the aristocracy and the wealthy. By contrast, the tradesmen surgeons only began to become respectable as a profession when they separated from their fellow barbers in the 18th century, and established surgery as an intellectual discipline under the influence of John Hunter and others. Only then did their status grow closer to that of physicians.[8] The lowliest category was the apothecaries. They established the right to treat the sick during the Plague of 1665, when the rich physicians and their equally rich patients moved out of London for their mutual safety.

The physicians and surgeons concentrated in the capital cities. They gave their services free to the new hospitals and dispensaries that were being established in Britain between 1700 and 1825 as charitable institutions for the sick poor. They made their living from the rich who were still cared for at home by a physician or by a combination of apothecary and physician.*

As the 19th century unfolded a clear pattern emerged. The growing number of specialists in London and the provincial cities earned their livelihood from private practice, but had established visiting rights at the voluntary hospitals that provided for those who could not afford to pay. The general practitioners looked after the growing middle classes and some of the poor in the expanding industrial towns. And Parliament established a third category of doctor when in 1872 local authorities were required to appoint medical officers of health. Under the Poor Law these doctors had specific responsibilities for the control of infectious diseases. That has become the speciality of public health medicine.

Between 1858 and 1900 an important division of labour known as 'the referral system' developed between general practitioners and specialists. It evolved first as an informal mechanism for limiting the effects of competition between the physicians and general practitioners, thus becoming embedded in professional etiquette. But structurally it split the profession. General practitioners were excluded from the care of patients in hospitals. Specialists were prevented from seeing patients directly – patients had to be referred. As Rosemary Stevens put it, 'The

---

* This division is neatly illustrated in the novel *Jane Eyre* by Charlotte Brontë. When Jane becomes ill, her aunt, Mrs Reed, sends for the apothecary. But Mrs Reed used a physician when she or her children needed medical attention.

physician and the surgeon retained the hospital, but the general practitioner retained the patient.'[8]

For the two groups there was mutual advantage. For the specialists it enabled them to concentrate even more on work in the hospitals. For general practitioners it secured their place as doctors of first contact in the community. For both it protected their incomes by reducing competition. Incomes were further protected by strict GMC rules on advertising by any doctor.

The term 'consultant' was a product of the referral system. At the beginning of the 20th century specialists were still few and far between, especially outside London. Their expertise was highly respected so that their opinions were sought by general practitioners on behalf of their patients. Literally these doctors were 'consulting' their expert colleagues.

In the first half of the 20th century specialisation continued apace. The new consultants tended to focus their energies not only on such treatment as existed but also particularly on accurate diagnosis. They needed the voluntary hospitals to take this work forward with the increasing facilities that they could provide, particularly where they were attached to universities. It was the basis of their teaching. So a pattern began to emerge in which the vocational driving force for the brightest and most able was in the domain of clinical problem solving and clinical description and research as intellectual challenges in their own right. Patients could thus be seen as merely a necessary vehicle for this activity rather than the primary focus.

In this period general practice was, by contrast, numerically and politically strong but intellectually weak. The Lloyd George National Insurance Act of 1911 provided state-insured healthcare for working men (but not for their families), and the beginnings of a more secure social and economic base, especially in the industrial areas of the north of England. General practitioners had no further training after qualification. The foundation medical degree was by common consent and by law all that was required to produce the basic doctor. They were taught by specialists who did not understand family practice because they had no experience of it other than as occasional locums in their youth. Most general practitioners were single-handed, working from their own homes. They tackled every problem that they thought lay within their competence. Some undertook surgery. Almost all attended confinements in women's own homes. They were regarded as inferior to consultants by patients and specialists alike because they were generalists, not experts. But the best of them became much respected in their communities for the care they provided. They were very accessible because they lived alongside their patients – the 'family doctor', like my father.

The tribe in the NHS

The NHS was introduced in 1948. It is a remarkable historical fact that, in its structure and organisation, it was built around the existing tribal divisions of the medical profession, based primarily on the referral system. It was a tripartite service. Specialists, who became salaried, saw the hospitals as their main base whilst retaining separate private practice. General practitioners acquired a registered list of patients in an evolutionary development of the panel and referral systems. They became independent contractors to the NHS. For the state, the gatekeeper role of the general practitioner would become the foremost instrument of cost containment. Public health medicine was embodied in the local authorities that had local public health responsibilities.

The new NHS was strapped for cash from the beginning. Demand greatly exceeded capacity from the very start. I remember the queues for false teeth and spectacles. And I remember my father describing the huge surge in demand for both primary and hospital care. For example, women in his practice who had awful prolapse – 'dropped womb' – for years now came forward to have them repaired. The politicians knew that rationing was inevitable – though they would not call it that – as a result of which an unwritten collusive understanding emerged between the state and the medical profession. The general practitioners would act as a first filter – the gatekeeper. They would deal with every problem they could, and would prioritise the problems they referred by degree of urgency. They would have an essentially protected monopoly of primary medical care in return. The consultants would prioritise referred cases on the basis of 'clinical need' as they defined it. Their instrument was the waiting list. Access to hospital care was politically highly sensitive. The politicians believed that the public would trust the doctors more than politicians to carry rationing out. They were right, as politicians have shown unwittingly by attempting to manipulate the waiting lists over the years, primarily for political ends. The price successive governments were willing to pay for all this was a huge measure of professional autonomy and freedom from scrutiny for all NHS doctors. This degree of freedom contrasted with the relatively stricter controls adopted by the state in countries like the USA where private practice predominated.

The consultants

The term 'consultant' was institutionalised by the new NHS to define specialists who had the ultimate clinical authority in their units and hospitals. Admission to these appointments was fiercely competitive, particularly in the popular specialities. College fellowship and membership examinations were pitched at a deliberately high standard to cream off the best. Only those who got through this hurdle were ultimately given definitive appointments. This narrow filtering was a peculiarly UK phenomenon, the product of the referral system. The entry gate to specialisation in continental Europe and the USA at the time was much broader, in keeping with their more open approach to specialisation.

Even within this, there was further professional demarcation in the form of distinction awards. Aneurin Bevan introduced this system at the start of the NHS to make the rewards for the best doctors as achievable in the NHS as they were in private practice. He wanted the best consultants to commit their expertise and time to the new NHS, hence his famous remark that to achieve that he 'stuffed their mouths with gold'.* In essence a consultant's income from the NHS was supplemented by further payments called merit awards, which came initially in three categories starting with the lowest, C awards, to the highest, A awards. For most of the life of the NHS these awards have been made in secret.† The intention was to maintain patient and general practitioner confidence that all consultants were of comparable ability. The fear was that if qualitative differences, which clearly existed, were made public, patients would want to be referred to 'the best', with obvious consequences for hospital units without award holders and the ability of non- or low-award holders to attract private patients.

Furthermore, by agreement with the state, the awards were determined by consultants themselves on the basis of peer review. In the formative early years the President of the RCP, Churchill's doctor, Lord Moran (known in the profession as 'Corkscrew Charlie') presided. So the people who were the ultimate arbiters of who got what were men at the top of their respective specialities, particularly the presidents of the medical Royal Colleges.

It was a remarkable system of closed patronage. Overall it achieved the primary purpose, but at a price. In particular, it too contributed strongly to the élitist culture at the top of British medicine that at that time was all pervasive, especially in London. A premium was placed on excellence in research. Closely allied with this was good clinical practice, as defined by consultants themselves, in which the focus was on the scientific and technical aspects of the medical consultation. Contributions to education and training were less valued. It was taken for granted that consultants would be instinctively good teachers – it went with the job, so

---

* Quoted in Brian Abel-Smith (1964) *The Hospitals 1800–1948*, Ch. 29.
† It is only recently that there has been any management or lay input, that the names of the award holders have been made public and that a proper periodic review of awards has been introduced.

there was no special preparation for it. Young doctors were deeply influenced by this culture because the top people in medicine were the dominant role models. Implicitly, junior doctors were expected to be deferential if they wanted to make progress. Rocking the boat, unless one was quite exceptional, was not the way to progress a career. The questioning of clinical decisions by juniors had to be especially carefully done – within unwritten rules of behaviour within clinical 'firms.' Whistle blowing was not seen as part of the medical ethic. On the contrary, speaking out against a colleague was considered 'not done' and indeed was listed by the GMC until quite recently as an ethical offence known as disparagement.

Within this tightly hierarchical structure, stresses and strains developed. The perpetual argument about 'sub-consultants', that is, specialists who had completed training but who were not considered good enough for a consultant post, flickered on for years. Known as Senior Hospital Medical Officers, they had lower salaries and were not eligible for merit awards. In fact many did much of the ordinary senior work in which, they complained (especially where their consultants were away doing other things), they too often had to carry the responsibilities of a consultant without the advantages.

To summarise, in the hospital service there was a general picture of progressive specialisation, a steeply pyramidal career structure, a system of closed patronage and the protection of clinical practice from outside scrutiny, other than by peers. The fact that UK consultants were cut off by the referral system from primary contact with patients added to the perception of them by many patients as remote, apparently able to work miracles and therefore godlike. The public was happy with this. In the 1950s right through until the 1990s the system was perceived by the vast majority of people to bring huge benefits – which it did. Criticisms were mainly of the NHS itself – long waiting lists, poorly equipped hospitals and the general structural deficiencies with which we are all too familiar today.

This was the culture in which medical students like myself were brought up. Specialisation represented success. Those who chose not to, or could not follow this highly competitive route were, as Lord Moran put it, deemed to have 'fallen off the ladder'. No thought was given by the establishment to what the consequences might be for the millions of patients who were looked after by so-called lesser doctors.

A grateful state, still chronically hard up, accepted all this. So the era of 'the Gods'* was born.

But it is important to add this: just as surely now the era of the gods has virtually gone. Over the years there has been a huge increase in

---

* As Jean Ritchie described them in her report on Rodney Ledward. See reference 77.

numbers of consultants in district and general hospitals. Recent genera-
tions of consultants, many of them women, have a far more open,
rounded, engaging approach to patients. Similarly, attitudes to teaching
are changing with more consultants now appreciating the value of real
educational professionalism. They are, not least, products of the society
that sets today's values. Sir Lancelot Spratt has become an anachronism, a
relic.

General practitioners

The situation in general practice at the start of the NHS could not have
been more different. In 1948 an Australian epidemiologist working at
Harvard, Joseph Collings, had reported extensively on the state of
general practice and its fitness as a provider of primary care in the new
NHS. He carried out an in-depth study of practice premises, equipment
and the general arrangements for care, the report occupying nearly half
an issue of the medical journal, the *Lancet*.[9] His conclusion was that
general practice was inadequate for the function expected of it, but that it
had potential if it could be rebuilt as a system of primary care.

Essentially the problem was lack of professional standards. General
practice consisted almost entirely of single-handed practice. There was
strong competition for patients, to a point where doctors' manners
seemed to matter more than their clinical competence, hence the saying
'You will never lose a patient through bad medicine.' By inference, you
could if you were ill-mannered.

At one extreme there was exceptionally good practice that offered
patients a very high standard of honest and competent care underpinned
by a strong sense of service. At the other were doctors who made no
effort to keep themselves up to date. As Collings found, their surgeries
were dirty and ill-equipped, their systems were poor, where these existed
at all, and their attitudes to patients were reflected in their minimalist
approach to service. In between these two extremes was a long line of
other practitioners who came somewhere in the middle. The result was
that many people got good care. But many did not.

The Collings Report produced a sharp professional reaction. The most
constructive outcome was the formation of a College of General Practitioners in 1952 – to set standards for general practice for the first time.
Only a small minority of general practitioners joined at the outset. My
father was a foundation member. However, many other practitioners
questioned the need for specific professional standards in general
practice. There was no consensus. Doctors defended what they saw as
their right to interpret the job as they thought fit – professional autonomy.

General practice survived in the new NHS by the skin of its teeth. It
was politically strong because of the near monopoly of primary care

created by the referral system. The new NHS needed cheap primary care to filter the huge volume of self-limiting or minor illness, and general practitioners were already providing some sort of service. General practitioners elected for a capitation system of payment* rather than a salary, as the specialists had done. The terms of their contract of service with the NHS were written very generally, requiring them only to do all those things that general practitioners are expected to do. The architects of the contract had left it so open for the best of reasons – to allow for changes as practice altered with new developments over time, without the need to resort regularly to Parliament. To general practitioners their 'independent contractor status' in the NHS was a prized possession. The practical effect, however, was to legitimise in contract a huge variation in the range of practice content and implicit clinical standards that was to bedevil general practice standards right up to the present day. It gave a contractual framework for unrestrained autonomy to continue. The British Medical Association (BMA) defended this 'right' with great energy each time the State chiselled away at the edges. What patients thought was never a serious consideration for either party. There were no well-organised patients' associations in those days.

When I entered general practice in 1960, morale was at rock bottom. Many UK-trained doctors were emigrating. A basic cause was insufficient investment to bring in the new group practice people were developing. This was being advocated and developed by leaders of the new College and by the government's own advisors, particularly the far-sighted Chief Medical Officer, Sir George Godber. Essentially the problem was with the way in which general practitioners were reimbursed for their expenses. When the NHS began, the BMA had secured an agreement that the NHS put into a 'pool' for the reimbursement of practice expenses all monies that had been spent; but, crucially, the money was to be shared equally amongst all doctors, irrespective of the expenses actually incurred by individuals. The effect of this was that general practitioners who invested minimally in their premises, staff and equipment made a profit at the expense of those who wanted to modernise their premises, buy new equipment and engage new staff. It was cottage industry versus the new group practices. For progressive doctors it was demoralising. Nevertheless many of us up and down the country dug into our pockets to modernise as best we could, not just for patients, but for our staff and ourselves.

However, the effort was not sustainable. In 1965 the progressive doctors, sick of being penalised as they saw it for investing in good care, revolted. I remember it vividly – I was one of them. In desperation we ousted the conservative BMA leadership, to replace them with leaders who were in tune with our new agenda. Then the BMA, thus redirected

---

* A basic fee for every patient registered.

and reinvigorated under the late James Cameron, did battle with the Wilson government, the outcome of which was a new charter for general practice.[10] The charter laid the foundation and provided the infrastructure for the modern team-based practice that the College had pioneered. It demonstrated that progressive doctors could achieve change by overcoming initial conservatism and inertia in both the BMA and the government.

But a better practice environment did not solve the problem of poor practice. The issues were essentially professional – standards and training. The new College introduced an examination for membership that tested the competencies needed for general practice. It pressed for proper vocational training being taught by people who practised the subject. This meant training in practices that, because of their reputation for providing good care and their interest in teaching, could provide the right environment and role model. The BMA supported this although many general practitioners were sceptical. But the BMA support was conditional on training remaining voluntary, which it did until 1982. Even when mandatory training came, eventually with BMA agreement, it took until the second half of the 1990s before there was a proper assessment of all completing training, so that patients would know that they were getting a fully-trained, competent doctor. Over the years the BMA had strenuously opposed the College's various attempts to bring this kind of rigour to the outcome of training, because of the concern of its activists that general practitioner trainees who failed a competence assessment should nevertheless be entitled to a full living as a general practitioner. Nine years of training should not go for naught. As we shall see later, this kind of conflict between public and professional interests would create real divisions and tensions in general practice and its institutions that have persisted until recent times.

Precisely because general practice had this problem of poor or unsafe practice, it provided at the same time a stimulus for the development of a kind not seen in specialist medicine. Before it could begin to deal with the albatross of poor practice, the new College had to cut the cord with specialist medicine and discover itself – what general practice was and what it should become. Thus the 1970s saw the leading edge of general practice in intellectual ferment.* The concept of 'whole-person' medicine,

---

* There were some remarkably talented people involved. For example, the late William Pickles, the late John Fry, Keith Hodgkin and Julian Tudor Hart described patterns of morbidity in the community for the first time. The late Paul Freeling analysed the content of consultations. The late EV Kuennsberg and Michael Drury pioneered teamwork and practice management. Clifford Kay led the first international study into the effects of the oral contraceptive pill. The late Patrick Byrne introduced new assessment methods to training. John Horder and Marshall Marinker led the development of small-group teaching. Brian Jarman devised his famous Index of Deprivation. Others are mentioned throughout my text.

the importance of interpersonal relationships and communications in the doctor–patient relationship and in clinical teamworking, and ideas about auditing the quality of care were being discussed and tested. Audio and videotaped consultations of doctors with patients were studied so that trainers and trainees could improve their bedside skills and manners. Some practitioners created patient participation groups in their practices. At the same time this part of general practice opened its doors and its mind to the outside world, as I described in Chapter 2 – that of education, the behavioural sciences, sociology and health services research in particular. So it benefited from the experience of people in these fields who offered new insights on medical practice. Equally it turned its attention overseas, to the USA and the old Commonwealth in particular, to bring in new ideas on medical education and the rapidly developing American expertise on quality assessment.

By the late 1970s, therefore, one element of general practice was beginning to evolve a professional culture in which relationships with patients' wants and needs were to the fore. That maximalist culture included attention to quality through standard setting and clinical audit. It was taken to its fullest in the teaching practice system, and so was to be hugely important in creating a culture of performance monitoring in general practice in the 1970s and 1980s. This would make the management of professional change when revalidation was proposed relatively straightforward for general practice because, at the end of the century, a substantial minority of general practitioners through their own experience understood broadly what was involved.

In general terms general practice was always weaker on the clinical diagnostic aspects of professionalism than were the hospital specialities and invariably stronger in the area of relationships with patients and communications. Specialists saw these as less important as they saw themselves primarily as technical experts to whom patients had been referred essentially for their technical professionalism. So the two main parts of medicine had things to offer each other if only they had the wit to do so, but regrettably their tribalism has prevented them from doing much of this until really quite recently. But now all sorts of bridges have been built, particularly in the education of all doctors.

Public health doctors

Public health medicine is the third main arm of the medical profession. The development of this branch was to be separate from the specialists and general practitioners from the earliest beginnings because of the decision by Parliament to base public health on the local authorities. They had responsibility for fever hospitals that were established to isolate patients with serious infections like diphtheria and scarlet fever, and sanatoriums that were introduced for patients with tuberculosis.

In the early years of the Poor Law, the public health overlap with general practitioners was substantial. Many general practitioners worked part time as medical officers of health. Most were public vaccinators. And there was a major complementary role in the notification and control of infectious diseases, which in the pre-antibiotic era were a serious cause of death and morbidity.

Public health medicine began to take shape as a speciality in its own right in the 1880s. In 1888 the newly introduced Diploma in Public Health became compulsory under the Local Government Act. Later, as the NHS was formed, public health medicine would be separated even further from the specialists and the general practitioners. This happened because of the political decision to base hospital services and general practice around their own specially created health authorities, leaving local government authorities with quite limited responsibilities in this area.

Culturally, this put public health medicine into its own tribal box. A few distinguished scientists developed a bridgehead for public health medicine in the universities. In the UK public health medicine continued to be medically dominated, quite unlike the situation in the USA where it became a multidisciplinary speciality at a much earlier stage.

Gender

Until relatively recently doctors were men, and undoubtedly this masculine emphasis has had an effect on the way in which the profession has developed. It was only towards the end of the 19th century that women were allowed in, and then only in penny numbers. A serious change in the intake of women into the profession did not really begin until the 1970s and 1980s. Today the proportion of female students is slightly higher than male and this is now beginning to be reflected in the career structure.

Within the profession women have been treated less equally than men until quite recently. Indeed there is still thought by some to be a 'glass ceiling' in some specialities, particularly surgery. Women, mainly because of child bearing, have tended to choose specialities that are perceived to be more flexible in their professional arrangements. So, for example, general practice, anaesthesia, public health medicine, psychiatry and community paediatrics are popular choices in this category.

Overseas-qualified doctors

Another significant element in the make-up of the medical profession is in the ethnic mix. Until the 1960s doctors working in Britain were largely qualified in the United Kingdom. Then an important inward migration of doctors who had qualified overseas began, the majority from the Indian subcontinent and elsewhere in the Commonwealth. At the same time, UK-trained doctors were emigrating to the old Commonwealth and the USA. So there is a picture of ebb and flow.

Many overseas-qualified doctors came for postgraduate training, and some of these had high expectations of a fulfilling career in the NHS. But for too many that was not to be. The pyramidal career structure in the specialities required more people to be in junior positions at the base of the pyramid than there were senior positions available. One consequence was that UK-qualified doctors tended to be selected for popular specialities, while overseas-qualified doctors tended to stay longer in specialist training, then enter a shortage speciality or drift into a sub-consultant appointment. Ultimately many would find their way into shortage areas in general practice. Unquestionably there has been racism in medicine. This very sensitive question was fully explored recently by Naaz Coker and her colleagues in an excellent King's Fund series of papers.[11] There were also, however, some important standards issues (*see* Chapter 5).

The tribe and the consumer

This then was the tribe that faced the consumer revolution of the 1980s. It was profoundly professional in its own terms, providing a much revered and valued service to a grateful and largely supportive community. The high status and affection felt by most patients for their doctors – general practitioners, specialists and the non-clinical doctors in public health – was borne of a recognition of the dedication, high order of skills, and the relationship between those who feel ill and those who have the power to cure or relieve suffering. Doctors and medicine had served society well, and society had accorded the medical profession the status and place that reflected the humanity of the service offered and the vulnerability of those who were aware of their need for it. It was a collusive relationship that reflected and encouraged the vocational basis of the medical profession. The downside was that it encouraged arrogance in some borne of highly intellectual and demanding training, and the positional superiority that offered. The profession was highly hierarchical in its training and career structure, status-ridden, white and male dominated.

It had a view of the patient–doctor relationship, encouraged and endorsed by the patient, that did not allow for the patient or their relatives to have much say. It had been a situation and relationship that had been in place for a long time.

For the medical profession therefore, the consequences of the election of Mrs Thatcher's government in 1978 were to be as profound as the election of Clement Attlee's government that had brought in the NHS. As Maurice Shock[4] had noted in 1994, the profession misread the signs. The majority of the profession missed the point that consumerism was coming to healthcare in the UK, carrying with it different public expectations of doctors and their accountability. In the light of the characteristics and history that I have described, that is hardly surprising. The partners in the collusion were developing at a different pace – society and patients moving out of respecting a profession and its practitioners simply by historical right and traditional relationships, leaving the doctors behind floundering in surprise.

So the profession went into aggressive mode against the NHS reforms instituted in the early 1990s. Early tactical successes against the government created a false sense of security against change. It was this, plus the ingrained belief in the overriding importance of providing relief from suffering as the touchstone of society's evaluation of professional worth, that prevented the profession from understanding and coming to terms with the implications of a different and less dominating role for the medical profession in its relationship with the public and the state.

We had therefore a combination of an understandably blinkered view of the profession's power and position in the overall order of the world, together with its lack of foresight as to its consequences when it came up against the new views on patient autonomy, accountability and transparency. These consequences were to hit the profession like an express train in the aftermath of Bristol.

4

Regulating the tribe, 1858–1970

What's so special about professions?

Professions in general

As I indicated in the last chapter, specialist medicine in the western world had an aura of invincibility in the fifties and sixties – it offered huge benefits to mankind and it alone knew how to deliver them. Behind this apparent invincibility lay the fundamental tenets of a profession.

Every occupation is subject to some kind of contract, some set of rules. However, professions over the years have claimed and obtained special recognition for their regulation, which set them apart from the rest of the world of craftsmen, tradesmen or artisans, or shopkeepers. Freidson,[12] describing the basis of self-regulation, said that the special privilege of freedom from control of outsiders or professional autonomy could be justified by three claims: 'First, there is such an unusual degree of skill and knowledge required in professional work that non-professionals are not equipped to evaluate or regulate it. Second, it is claimed that professionals are responsible – that they may be trusted to work conscientiously without supervision. And third, the profession itself may be trusted to take the proper regulatory action on those rare occasions when an individual does not perform his work competently or ethically.' He argued that a profession is the sole source of competence both to recognise deviant performance, and also ethical enough to control it – to regulate itself in general. In this way the autonomy of a profession is justified by the fact that it regulates itself.

This relationship between society and the profession has been described as a 'regulative bargain' by Stacey.[13] Such a bargain, she said, carries with it advantages for the occupation, which include autonomy in the workplace, a near monopoly of the market, the facility to regulate the terms and conditions of work and the control of the education required for practice. In return for these formidable privileges, the profession promises that all those who carry the title shall be competent and trustworthy, such that they may be approached with confidence by potential clients and that they will regulate themselves to this end. That regulation involves ensuring that only those who enter the profession are appropriately trained and educated, and that those who deviate from the standards of the profession shall be disciplined and removed from the profession, if necessary.

Medicine in particular

Medicine, because of its complexity, is a profession for whom these criteria apply pre-eminently. The Merrison Committee Inquiry in 1975 into the regulation of the medical profession set out the position succinctly.[14] It said: 'An instructive way of looking at regulation is to see it as a contract between public and profession, by which the public go to the profession for medical treatment because the medical profession has made sure it will provide satisfactory treatment. Such a contract has the characteristics of all freely made contracts – mutual advantage.' The key instrument of regulation is the register of those appropriately qualified. Any such register, Merrison asserted, if it is not to be a fraud on the public, must list only those who have a certain standard of competence.

It is important to distinguish between self-regulation as applied to the individual, and collective self-regulation by the profession as a group. In medicine, a doctor's highly developed sense of personal self-discipline is vital to patients. Stripped of everything else, the key element in medicine is the highly individualistic nature of clinical decision making I described in the last chapter. There are no conceivable circumstances in which the myriad of individual decisions taken by doctors could be closely supervised. So the patient consulting a doctor at any moment in time is dependent on that doctor's conscientiousness in practising within the limits of their competence. Knowledge, skill, self-awareness, integrity and conscience are the key attributes that go with effective personal self-regulation. They are the starting point for establishing a relationship of trust.

The problems arise in the collective self-regulation of a profession. Theoretically the medical profession, sure of its science and its technical know-how, should be better placed than any outside groups to define what for it should be best, acceptable and unacceptable practice. It ought to be able to sustain a high level of integrity. But, as the critics of collective self-regulation argue, there is the danger that self-interest can override these ideals. The need to regulate aberrant behaviour effectively can conflict with the natural solidarity of those who share a professional interest – usually resolved in the public mind as doctors 'looking after their own.' 'Misplaced collegiality'[15] can undermine effective collective self-regulation.

To complicate matters further, medicine today is vastly more complex and demanding than it ever was. It requires clinical teamworking on an unprecedented scale. That in turn implies a degree of collective responsibility for the observance of professional standards at the workplace, because the outcomes for the patient are now very often the product of contributions from more than one member of the profession, and often from members of several professions together. Indeed it is at the level of the clinical team that there is a natural meeting point where professional and managerial systems of regulation come together in what is now called clinical governance.

The net effect of these developments, that were brought into such sharp focus at Bristol, has resulted in a rethinking by government, the professions and the public about the basic nature of modern regulation in healthcare. One outcome has been apparently to dilute the importance of professional regulation itself, seeing it merely as part of a wider, joined-up system. But, paradoxically, these very same developments have placed an even higher duty on each profession and its regulatory body to make sure its contribution to the regulatory framework works effectively. Patients want to be sure of their individual doctor as well as the system and will not in future forgive a profession that does not ensure this.

Over the last ten years these conflicting tensions have played out, until a different form of professionally led regulation emerged. This was partly as a result of a changing power relationship between the patient and the doctor in favour of the patient. It was partly because of society's insistence that professional regulation must be able to deliver and be accountable outside the profession, particularly in the aftermath of Bristol and the other high-profile cases of the 1990s. To get the proper perspective, we need to look at the foundations that lie in the specifics of medical regulation.

The regulators

Professional self-regulation

For most people the GMC is the definitive body that should protect them from poor or dangerous practice. The public sees the GMC as the key to the proper accountability of doctors because it is the statutory regulator. Its stewardship of the Medical Register is the basis of its power – it registers doctors, thus entitling them to practise in the UK. By definition, the body controlling the Register decides what precisely registration stands for. As Merrison put it, 'This power is obvious enough in relation to the individual doctor who is prevented from practising because of his professional misconduct. More significant is the power to place a name on the Register because it is this power which is at the route of the GMC's power over educational institutions.'[14] The GMC, through its control of the Register, validates qualifications from universities and other professional bodies by recognising them for registration. In summary then the GMC licenses doctors to practise in the UK through registration. It sets general standards of professional competence and conduct. It controls the entry to medicine and the training of medical students at university. It disciplines doctors who behave badly. Theoretically at least it should underpin all facets of professional regulation by virtue of its primary responsibilities as the licensing body. Understandably, doctors are wary of it. It is associated with trouble and punishment, which is why the medical profession has always been ambivalent about the GMC. I felt the same wariness when I was a medical student and a young doctor.

All doctors now undergo some form of postgraduate training. Two additional regulators have had responsibility for supervising the content and quality, and of certificating doctors who complete this training satisfactorily. The Joint Committee on Postgraduate Training for General Practitioners (JCPTGP) does this for general practice, and the Specialist Training Authority (STA) for the specialists. Under the government's modernisation plans the two bodies are to be replaced by the Postgraduate Medical Education and Training Board that will combine their functions. The names of certificated doctors are placed on the Specialist Register held by the GMC. A comparable register is planned for general practice. So it is the GMC that is ultimately responsible for the integrity of these registers.

But the GMC and the certificating bodies are not the only regulators. The medical profession has, additionally, non-statutory institutions that have a very important role in professional regulation. Thus the medical Royal Colleges are charitable organisations that have the object of setting professional standards for their own specialities. They determine the nature of specialist training and accredit training posts. They conduct examinations. They work closely with the specialist societies that are the ultimate repositories of expertise in the subspecialities of medicine.

The BMA is a national professional association and registered trade union. It works through major craft committees representing the main medical tribes – general practice, the hospital specialities, public health medicine, academic doctors and junior doctors. But because the collegiate structure evolved before the BMA was founded, the medical Royal Colleges have retained effective control of their speciality standards and the BMA carries out its representative role within that framework.

However that has not been the case in general practice, where the BMA has been historically and practically the dominant force. Here there has been a real tension between the RCGP, as a voluntary membership organisation that can advocate the high standards set and achieved by its members, and a BMA General Practitioner Committee that has responsibility to represent the whole of general practice, from the highest idealists to those working to bare minimum standards.

Regulation by contract

However, regulation through professional machinery is only part of the picture. In the UK, since the inception of the NHS, we have had massive professional regulation by contract in addition to statutory regulation by the GMC. Governments or their agents have centrally determined doctors' contracts. The BMA, as the registered trade union of doctors, has secured for itself the sole right to negotiate for the medical profession.* All sorts of professional issues have been negotiated through this route. For example, the whole of general practice training has been underpinned by NHS legislation. Both general practitioner and consultant contracts have become increasingly specific about the nature of doctors' work, and require such professional activities as appraisal and clinical audit. Complaints about doctors have been normally handled in the vast majority of cases through government arrangements that have been operated by NHS management with significant input from the BMA.

Of the two parties involved in both the licensure and employment contract dimensions – the government and the medical profession – the doctors have until now been dominant. The state as employer has until recently been less than assertive in protecting patients' interests and as we shall see has been party to some very unsatisfactory compromises on standards of practice. The licensing body, the GMC, was unwilling until recently to step into the arena of poorly performing doctors, because of the tendency of both governments and the BMA to try and settle concerns through contract, which of course largely excluded the public. The operation of these two systems, side by side, but with no real co-ordination, has been one of the factors contributing to the delay in taking effective action on poorly performing doctors.

Against that general background I will describe the origins of the GMC, and the events that led in the 1970s to the first major revision of its functions, and the pressure from within for it to take on its responsibilities for managing poorly performing doctors.

* However, PMS pilots are outside the central negotiating machinery; and the impact of the BMA's failure in England to convince the consultants and junior doctors of the acceptability of the new Consultants' Contract in November 2002 has yet to be seen.

The GMC, 1858–1950

The General Medical Education and Registration Council of the United Kingdom (shortened to 'GMC' in 1951) was created by the Medical Act of 1858. As the GMC pointed out later,[16] the Act was passed 'largely as a result of initiative within the profession, and the establishment of the Council (GMC) was desired as much for the protection of the duly qualified medical practitioner as for the protection of the public'. Pyke-Lees (a former GMC registrar) points to the 'deep-felt necessity for a radical improvement in the education of the main body of medical practitioners'[17] at the time, hence the emphasis on education.

But there was also the need to establish reciprocity of professional privileges in the three divisions of the United Kingdom. Prior to 1858 there had been 19 separate licensing bodies.[5] So for instance a practitioner with an Edinburgh licence would be unable to extend his practice legally to London or Dublin or indeed even Glasgow! This clutter of local qualifications, and the inadequate tests required for many of them, when coupled with the large number of wholly unqualified practitioners, made it impossible for the public to distinguish the qualified from the unqualified. Indeed, estimates based on the census returns of 1841 suggest that nearly 5000 of the 15 000 practitioners then practising in England were unqualified.

The composition of the first Council, the subject of much lobbying with Parliament, emerged finally as consisting of 24 members, who with the exception of six who were nominated by the Privy Council represented the medical Royal Colleges and universities. General practitioners had no places. As Stacey[5] pointed out, the medical Royal Colleges had avoided, for the time being at least, the curtailment of their powers, which the wide-ranging authority that was originally proposed would have imposed. Lord Richardson, a later President, described the powers of the Council as 'slender and vaguely expressed . . . and it was hard for it to assert its authority, which was opposed by those well-established institutions that were represented upon it. . . . The opposition was especially difficult as it was both without and within the Council.'[18]

How prophetic Richardson's words have turned out to be. For the limits and the scope of the Council have been determined over the years to a very large extent by what the institutions of medicine – initially the medical Royal Colleges and the universities, and later the BMA – would allow it to do. Indeed this pattern of behaviour only ended with the Bristol case when the GMC began to act more unequivocally in the public interest, even at the cost of incurring the wrath of the BMA.

The constitution of the Council was amended in 1886. Five practitioners were to be elected to the Council by postal vote of the profession as a whole because the profession considered the first Council to be unrepresentative, especially of general practitioners who at that time constituted by far the majority of doctors. Under this Act the educational powers of the Council were strengthened so that, for the first time, applicants for registration had to have passed examinations in medicine, surgery and midwifery. It was this Act that empowered the Council to appoint inspectors in order to attend the final or qualifying examinations in medicine. The Council, if it was not satisfied with the standard of proficiency expected and revealed, was empowered to make appropriate representations to the Privy Council, which had the power to withdraw recognition of an educational body.

Interestingly, the Act did not give registered medical practitioners an absolute right of entitlement to practise medicine. So it was – and still is – possible for any citizen to carry out any medical intervention. Anyone can ask a friend to take their appendix out – quite legally – provided that the friend does not claim to be a doctor and the person is willing. But what the Act did do was to create a virtually reserved title by embodying in statute functions and privileges that could only be carried out or exercised by a registered medical practitioner. So, for example, only registered medical practitioners could certify statutory documents; only they could be included on a medical list or panel under the National Health Insurance Act 1911 and so on.

In addition to the function of keeping a register of practitioners, and of controlling basic medical education, the new Council was also concerned with professional discipline. In those early years cases brought before the Council were mainly concerned with such matters as fraudulent registration and infamous conduct such as 'keeping an anatomical museum containing waxworks of a disgusting character'.[17] Interestingly, in 1889 the President commended to the qualifying bodies (who supervised the medical qualifications of the day) that they exercise independent disciplinary action against their licentiates, after which the GMC could act. Pyke-Lees reported that between 1858 and 1886 the GMC took such consequential action following disciplinary action by a licensing body in no fewer than 23 cases, while in the same period 26 practitioners were erased by the Council for convictions or for infamous conduct in a professional respect. The Council, in the words of its President in 1889, was concerned 'that it should not seem over-anxious to be at work' since 'the spreading abroad of the shortcomings of any erring members of our honourable profession is a proceeding to be carefully restrained within precise limits'.[17]

In today's language that sounds like protectionism! Little wonder then that George Bernard Shaw wrote of the professions as 'all conspiracies against the laity'[19] and was particularly scathing about doctors. In his preface on doctors in *The Doctor's Dilemma*, there is a postscript dated 1930.[20] In this he refers to 'the need for bringing the medical profession under responsible and effective public control'. This was a development that he thought had become 'constantly more pressing as the inevitable collisions between the march of discovery in therapeutic science and the *reactionary obsolescence* [my italics] of the General Medical Council have become more frequent and sensational'. He added, by way of a further postscript in 1933, 'The condition of the medical profession is now so scandalous that unregistered practitioners* obtain higher fees and are more popular with educated patients than registered ones.' So that is how he perceived the value to the public of GMC registration in the inter-war years.

The Medical Acts of 1950 and 1956

The lay role

The Medical Act of 1950 made important changes to the constitution of the GMC, to its disciplinary functions and medical education. The number of members was increased to 47 with eight crown nominees, including laymen. This inclusion of laymen dates back to 1926, since when it had been the practice of the Privy Council to include one layman among the five people nominated to the Council. According to Pyke-Lees,[17] George Bernard Shaw claimed some of the credit for the original intention of having lay members. Lay members were members of the public who were charged with maintaining a critical vigilance over the Council, especially in matters of discipline, and should 'represent the consumer interest'. Shaw maintained his scepticism: 'Until the General Medical Council is composed of hard-working representatives of the suffering public, with doctors who live by private practice rigidly excluded except as assessors, we shall still be decimated by the vested interest of the private side of the profession in disease.'[20]

Educating doctors: a new start

The 1950 Act also introduced the pre-registration year, which was recognition of the fact that, after qualification, a period of one year's supervised apprenticeship should be a requirement for every doctor. This fairly modest change was built on in 1968 when a Royal Commission on Medical Education,[21] chaired by Lord Todd, reported on the future development of education for doctors. It was the significant regulatory event of the 1960s.

The Commission really set medical education in a new direction, essentially to bring it into line with the rapidly developing science and

---

* Complementary practitioners in today's language.

practice of the subject itself. With full GMC support, the Todd Report made clear that the current undergraduate curriculum was not the way to produce safe and competent general practitioners. General practice, as both the RCGP and the BMA had recognised, should have its own training. Given this, it would be possible to reconstruct basic medical education on more modern lines, as a generic preparation for later specialist training rather than as an end in itself. As a corollary, the report proposed vocational training registration on completion of specialist training and vocational training for general practitioners.

Interestingly, the potentially biggest change was to the London medical schools. The Commission recommended a reduction in the number of London schools from 12 to six, with each to be integrated as the faculty of medicine in a multidisciplinary university institution. That did not happen then. It was Virginia Bottomley, Secretary of State for Health some 30 years later, who finally and successfully gripped this hot potato.*

And so the 1960s brought to a close a quiet century of regulation for the profession. Bernard Shaw apart, it had no great critics. But that was about to change.

---

* This was following the report she commissioned from Sir Bernard Tomlinson into the free-standing and postgraduate medical schools in London.

Part 2
Snakes and ladders

5

Lost opportunities, 1970–80

The swinging sixties were confident years in the country and the NHS, but the seventies were a different story. There was the oil crisis with its devastating effect on the economy, the miners' strike and the three-day week. In terms of financial investment, these had severe repercussions on the NHS. At the same time, medical discovery proceeded inexorably, pushing up the costs of care. The consultants challenged minister Barbara Castle over private practice. In 1974, a major NHS reorganisation ended the tripartite structure of the NHS. It introduced new management structures, not altogether successfully. It gave non-teaching hospitals a fairer deal and attempted to correct inequalities in the distribution of resources between regions. This was also a period of serious turbulence in the regulation of doctors, for the medical profession lost its confidence in the GMC.

It was not all doom and gloom. Geoffrey Rivett[22] describes this period as 'rethinking the NHS', as arguments and assumptions about the NHS were changing. Interest was growing within the profession for medical audit, stimulated in the USA by the creative thinking and method development for assessing and assuring healthcare quality. I caught the quality bug then.

Harbingers of change

I want to return to the situation in general practice, as it was there that new ideas about professionalism were emerging and the problems of poor practice were being recognised. In the 1970s there were four significant developments, all within the framework of the new vocational training for general practitioners. They were the harbingers of change in medicine generally.

First, we decided through the RCGP to professionalise teaching. We strengthened apprenticeship by adopting modern teaching methods, proper assessment and investing heavily in the professionalisation of doctors as teachers. Marshall Marinker, an exceptional general practitioner, established the London Teachers Workshops that became the prototype for other groups all over the country. The College, with the support of the Nuffield Trust, ran a series of inspirational 'Nuffield' courses for developing future leaders. All in all, teaching in general practice became a sought-after, high-status activity, so in the main compliance with the new practice standards was high. This was in contrast to the time trainees spent as senior house officers in hospital, where in the 1970s and 1980s the quality of supervision and teaching was highly variable.

Second, as I indicated in Chapter 2, as part of that professionalisation, we decided that trainees should be placed only in the best practices available to ensure they were exposed to good care.*[23] Role modelling was seen as crucial in developing professional attitudes and behaviours. From this decision grew the teaching practice system used throughout general practice today. The system was designed around explicit criteria and standards defining both the clinical and teaching qualities expected of a general practitioner trainer, and the practice environment considered suitable for patient care and learning. It was expected that teaching practices would demonstrate their compliance with these standards. Teaching contracts with the university postgraduate organisations were renewable on the basis of performance reviewed, usually at five-yearly intervals by the trainer's peers. The university postgraduate organisations were themselves subject to external inspection initially by the RCGP and later by the JCPTGP. Essentially training practice contracts were managed by the regional organisations and were accredited against national standards, often supplemented by local additions. The JCPTGP quality assured the regional process by periodic visits that included site visits to sample practices. Trainees (now called registrars) were regarded as colleagues and, in a sense, customers. So from the outset they were involved in the planning of their training, asked about their satisfaction with their training experience and took part in the review of their teachers. The vast majority of trainees found that this approach to training contrasted quite sharply with their experience in hospital posts where the relationships between juniors and consultants were more hierarchical.

* The National Trainee Practitioner Scheme had been set up previously, under the auspices of the NHS and the BMA. In the early sixties it failed. Recruitment slumped. An important cause was the huge variation in the quality of the learning experience, reflecting the variability in the attitudes and practices of trainers. Essentially there was no curriculum and no quality control.

Thirdly, the College commissioned six of us,* led by two outstanding general practitioners, John Horder and the late Patrick Byrne, to take a completely fresh look at the work of the general practitioner and the clinical task, to see if these could be described as a coherent whole. The result was the book *The Future General Practitioner: learning and teaching*.[24] It provided the intellectual basis for the discipline from which were derived the attributes of a good general practitioner.† For the first time we were clear what kind of doctor we were trying to produce, what were the basic qualities such a doctor should possess and therefore what should be taught and assessed. It became, and still is, the basis of our training in general practice.

Fourth, alongside this, medical audit was introduced experimentally. I have mentioned an example of an early audit group in my own region (Chapter 2). Doctors were starting to write up simple practice audits. In the mid-seventies the RCGP, through Donald Crombie, started to offer members a practice activity service. On a series of topics, of which referrals to specialists and home-visiting patients were examples, doctors gave the College their data. These data were then compared to data from others, and the results showing where one stood in relation to peers was fed back. That feedback was the starting point for asking questions.

This all went well as a voluntary effort. In 1982 the BMA and government were persuaded to make training mandatory, as the Todd Report had recommended. However, we failed as a College to persuade them that doctors completing training and entering NHS practices as principals should be tested at that point for their competence. Between 1975 and 1982, my colleagues and I in the Northern Region ran a regional certification system based on a combination of the membership examination of the RCGP (MRCGP) and regular assessments of doctors at work, because we thought that was an effective way of ensuring that trainees were ready for unsupervised practice. However, we could not sustain this against political pressure when training became mandatory in 1982. When the chips were down professional union power was too strong and the NHS was not yet prepared to challenge that. So we had a situation where, for many years, doctors entering general practice as principals had first to complete a course of training, but they could choose whether or not to have their competence on completion assessed by, for instance, taking the RCGP membership examination. So there was no way that the NHS, which was the contracting authority, could know whether those

---

* Dr John Horder, Chairman, Professor Patrick Byrne, Professor Paul Freeling, Professor Conrad Harris, Professor Marshall Marinker and myself.
† These attributes were later taken and modified by the GMC, and published in its 1987 guidance on specialist training. The GMC would later use this as part of its starting point for new standards for medicine – *Good Medical Practice*. I was involved in all three projects.

who chose not to be assessed were competent or not. The fact that many did so choose was reassuring, but for the patients of doctors who refused assessment it was more of a lottery and, for some, unsafe.

Consequently, it was inevitable that outside the training system huge variations in the quality of practice as a whole persisted. In my William Pickles lecture at the RCGP in 1975,[25] I pointed out that general practice, for all the improvements that had recently taken place, was still unwilling 'to agree minimum clinical and operational standards for all doctors, not just those who want them'. The RCGP, of which I was then Honorary Secretary, described the situation in 1977[26] in its evidence to the Royal Commission on the NHS as 'our main liability: poor care'. The picture of the assets of general practice must be balanced, the College said, by 'the frank recognition that care by some doctors is mediocre, and by a minority is of an unacceptably low standard'. Incompetence, failure to communicate, bad records, badly run appointment systems and poor deputising arrangements were cited as the main problems.

The RCGP position contrasted starkly with the stance of the BMA's General Medical Services Committee (GMSC) that represented general practice. Whilst the GMSC applauded doctors who were trying to provide good patient care, it rationalised its position about the anarchic state of poor care in the now infamous words of the late James Cameron, its Chairman, who frequently said, 'There is no such thing as a bad general practitioner.' The BMA lived to regret that. Cameron, who I knew as a good doctor,* saw this approach as the only way of keeping his committee together, of maintaining professional solidarity and therefore of not splitting general practice. Misplaced collegiality again.

In these clashes over standards of competence and patient safety, the Department of Health (DoH) and government expressed concern, but were not anxious enough to face up to the BMA. 'The profession regulates itself' was the cop-out for ministers and officials.

And in all this the GMC, the ultimate guardian of the standards, simply did not want to know. In the College Council we were immensely disappointed in it. We thought it should have been the body above all that would support us – and patients – over the standards/competence disputes with the BMA and the government.

The rebellion

The early 1970s saw the seeds of the rebellion in the profession about the GMC. The flashpoint was its unrepresentativeness. However different groups had different issues, but there was much common ground.

---

* James Cameron had led the modernising GP Charter negotiations.

General practice

At the time the RCGP's views of the GMC were sharply critical. I have explained the lack of GMC support on the poor practice issue. But there was more. The GMC was doing nothing about building primary care into the undergraduate curriculum even though it had signed up to this. And the RCGP, alone of all of the medical Royal Colleges, had no seat on the GMC, and the GMC was being difficult about this. All fuel for the College's exasperation. This was revealed in the evidence[27] the College gave later in 1973 to the Committee of Inquiry into the Regulation of the Medical Profession – the Merrison Committee. The tone of the College's evidence was indicative of the mood. The College described the GMC as 'isolated . . . and out of touch with the important developments in education and service.'

In line with the developments in general practice which I described above, we wanted vocational training for general practice to be mandatory, for specialist registration to be introduced as the Todd Commission had proposed. We also wanted the GMC to recognise the MRCGP examination as the proper test of competence on completion of training.* We were critical of the GMC's failure to implement its own 1967 recommendations to medical schools on undergraduate training and equally critical of the pre-registration year which we thought was a 'no man's land' between qualification and specialist training. We wanted all doctors to be regulated by a tougher, more broadly constituted GMC, new arrangements for sick doctors and a test of medical knowledge and of the English language for all doctors from overseas who wanted to practise in the UK. We wanted a GMC that would act like a purposeful regulator. To this end we thought that the GMC should 'be required to . . . find out to what extent its recommendations are heeded and report its findings to the public and the profession in annual and special reports'. We thought it should be 'required to challenge effectively universities and postgraduate organisations which continue to dissent from its recommendations'. The words 'required to' expressed our dissatisfaction and frustration with its unwillingness or inability – who can say which – to enforce its own policies.

On the specific issue of competence, we gave the Merrison Committee the published results from three recent MRCGP examinations, in which the candidates were obviously drawn only from a group of practitioners who had chosen to be assessed: 188 out of 289 passed, that is a 65% pass rate. The College went on to make a number of observations that derived from these data. Doctors who had completed vocational training had a

* It became a registerable qualification in 1976.

higher pass rate than newly appointed principals in the NHS who had qualified in the UK, but who had entered general practice without any vocational training. Doctors who had graduated overseas (excluding Eire) achieved a significantly lower pass rate. There was concern about doctors who failed badly, irrespective of their place of qualification. The College said, 'Further analysis has shown that most of these principals appointed in the NHS have shortcomings so fundamental that their safety as clinicians in unsupervised general practice must be questioned.' This evidence was published.* The issue for the College was simply this. Doctors wanting to practise as unsupervised principals in general practice should first complete vocational training, and on completion they should pass an assessment of competence. We could hardly have been plainer about the patient safety issue.

I have taken some time over the RCGP's views because in 1973 it expressed clearly that in some important respects the GMC was not protecting the public. Nor, as I showed earlier, was the NHS. Moreover, the GMC was not acting as we thought it should to implement its own (very good) recommendations on undergraduate training. This was not because it did not know what to do but because it lacked the will (and the sense of public duty) to require compliance, to stand up to vested interests in the profession, which wanted no change.†

Other areas of concern

The much-expanded establishment of medical specialists was also discontented, for different reasons. Margaret Stacey summarised these.[5] The new regional consultants in the NHS felt that their interests were not properly represented nationally and junior doctors were discontented about their pay and conditions of work. Much of this discontent flowed through the BMA where there was a feeling that the BMA leadership did not have the rank and file interests at heart. They were seen to be effectively part of the medical establishment. In addition the Todd Report proposed to extend the role of the GMC to 'specify in broad terms, and constantly keep under review, the professional training, experience and qualifications necessary to achieve recognised competence to exercise independent clinical judgement in a speciality.' This represented a direct threat to the power and autonomy of the Royal Medical Colleges, and was being resisted.

---

* The College later furnished Merrison and the GMC with consolidated figures for 1972–74, and later the GMC with the figures for 1975. The picture remained true.
† Yet despite the subsequent Merrison recommendations, it was 18 years before the GMC actually confronted the medical schools about the undergraduate curriculum, and 23 years before it got really serious about sorting out the pre-registration year.

In the 1960s there had been also growing concern within the GMC itself and the profession about how to handle doctors who were not fit to practise because of ill-health – usually mental illness, excessive alcohol use or the use of drugs. The disciplinary powers were the only instruments that the Council had. I served for a while as the Chairman of the Northumberland Local Medical Committee (LMC) in the 1960s, and I had personal experience of the problems this involved. I remember going opportunistically to persuade a colleague to resign from the NHS on grounds of his genuine ill health, which was potentially endangering his patients. With difficulty I was eventually successful. I would never have dreamt of telling the GMC as in no way could this doctor be considered as being guilty of serious professional misconduct, the only way the GMC had then of dealing with sick doctors. I remember how other doctors and I felt about having a colleague labelled as 'bad' when they were in reality 'sick doctors', and there was a concern therefore that this problem was seriously under-reported. This was the climate at around the time that Harold Shipman's drug abuse came to the attention of the GMC.

Margaret Stacey records that in the GMC the volume of work was rising inexorably because of the very success of medicine and the number of doctors practising in the health services. This and its impact on the logistics of registration alone made it impossible to operate the GMC on the income it derived from the single registration fee doctors paid on first being registered. So in responding to these problems the GMC took forward new proposals for legislation – the 1969 Bill – which amongst other things would have given it the power for the first time to levy an annual subscription for registration as a doctor – an annual retention fee. This would affect the pocket of every doctor and was the spark that ignited the fire-storm – money, as is so often the case, being the last straw!

Between 1970 and 1972 there followed a serious battle between an entrenched GMC and its President, the BMA and much of the medical profession. The core of the matter, for the profession, was the perceived and actual lack of adequate representation, particularly of general practitioners – 'no taxation without representation' was how doctors saw it. The BMA raised the political temperature by calling special representative meetings, and threatening withdrawal altogether from medical regulation through the GMC.

Matters came to a head in November 1972 when the GMC voted to go ahead with striking off dissident doctors who had not paid their retainer fees, all of them having already been repeatedly warned of this possibility. Lord Cohen and the Council took the view that it was unreasonable for those doctors who agreed to the retention fee to be subsidising those who chose not to. The Government was faced with the possibility that huge numbers of doctors would be removed from the Medical Register. It had to act, and so it took what was to be one of the most significant steps in the development of the regulation of the medical profession – it set up the Merrison Committee.

The Committee was appointed in November 1972 by Sir Keith Joseph, the Secretary of State for Health.[28] Its terms of reference were:

> to consider what changes need to be made in the existing provisions for the regulation of the medical profession; what functions should be assigned to the body charged with the responsibility for its regulation and how that body should be constituted to enable it to discharge its functions most effectively; and to make recommendations.

The role of professional self-regulation itself was not an issue. Sir Keith Joseph himself ruled that out when he added that 'the General Medical Council is a body with a notable record of service to the public and to the profession. It is not contemplated that the profession should be regulated otherwise than by a predominantly professional body . . .'

The Merrison Inquiry, 1972–75

Dr Alec Merrison, the Chairman, was a nuclear physicist and Vice-Chancellor of Bristol University. There were 15 members of the Merrison Committee altogether, of who seven were medical. The RCGP had proposed that I should be one of the two general practitioners on the Committee. The other general practitioner, Brian Whowell, was put forward by the BMA.

I remember that by far the best evidence was given by the GMC itself. By this time Sir John Richardson, a physician at St Thomas' Hospital, with an excellent mind and a somewhat healthy scepticism of his own college (RCP), was President. As the evidence taking proceeded, I remember Merrison saying to us one morning, 'All we have to do is sit here and wait for them all. They are working it out.' The focus provided by the mere presence of the inquiry was sufficient to get minds engaged, shorten time-scales and speed up developments already in progress. The pressure of the Bristol Public Inquiry later had the same effect. It concentrated minds.

And what of the results of Merrison?[14] Given the background of a profession that believed that no fundamental change was necessary within itself, and was generally sceptical about quality assurance, the recommendations for all their imperfections and omissions represented a major step forward. They are important to my story in terms of advancing the concept of professionalism in medicine. The Committee said that regulation should be largely self-directed because, in its view, it was 'in no doubt that the most effective safeguard for the public is the self-respect of the profession itself and that we should do everything to foster this self-respect'.[14] How that was interpreted was crucial to what happened at Bristol and in other cases.

One of the main thrusts of the report and recommendations was about medical education. Building on the Todd Commission of the previous decade, Merrison recommended a two-tier structure of registration. There should be a restrictive general register, setting out who could be a doctor, and a new indicative specialist register which would indicate those who have satisfactorily completed specialist training and, in due course, the new training for general practice. There were specific recommendations about improving early postgraduate education after qualification, in particular for re-badging and improving the quality of the pre-registration year for which the GMC was responsible.

The Committee considered evidence about overseas-qualified doctors. In its evidence on this the GMC told the Committee:[14]

> Indirectly the decisions of the Council in this area have, at least in recent years, been to some extent influenced by medical manpower requirements. In the first place the medical manpower needs of the NHS have caused the rapid growth in the volume of applications for full, provisional and temporary registration by overseas doctors, which has occurred in the last 20 years. In granting temporary registration, therefore, where the doctor has to be selected for employment before he can apply, the Council has been responding to the manpower needs of the health service. Secondly, in approaching the question of the possible withdrawal of recognition from qualifications previously recognised, the Council has been aware that any precipitate action might embarrass the NHS; and that this factor might influence the Privy Council in deciding any appeal against a refusal by the Council to recognise or continue to recognise a qualification.

The health departments were matter of fact in their evidence. They said, 'The arrangements for the admission of overseas doctors must neither impede nor deter those whose medical education and ability are of an appropriate standard and character for work in the NHS.'[14] The Committee concluded that this differed little, if at all, from 'an assertion that the NHS should set its own standards', according to the manpower availability of the day. The Committee fundamentally disagreed with this view because it meant that in times of doctor shortage, the standards required for medical practice could be watered down.

In the event the Committee came to 'the inescapable conclusion . . . that there are substantial numbers of overseas doctors whose skill and care . . . fall below that generally acceptable in this country, and it is possible that there are some who should not have been registered'. As to cause, the Committee believed that 'this unsatisfactory situation is principally to be attributed to a willingness on the part of the GMC to allow its duty as the protector of medical standards to be compromised by the manpower requirements of the NHS'.[14]

However, it rejected the recommendation put forward by the RCGP and some others that doctors coming from any country outside the UK should have their knowledge and linguistic competence tested before being registered, just as the Americans were doing with their ECFMG* examination.† Instead, it adopted the GMC's recommendations, namely, the restriction of recognition as a route to full registration, the replacement of temporary by limited registration and the imposition of clinical and linguistic tests upon those applying for the new limited registration. It recommended that ways should be worked out whereby overseas-trained doctors could apply for the proposed new specialist registration. And it recommended that the DoH should think about a training programme for doctors from overseas, seeing presciently that the European Economic Community (EEC) was a likely future area of difficulty.

The issue of re-certification and/or re-licensure (later to be called revalidation) was discussed and discarded as being too difficult: 'The introduction of re-licensure schemes would represent an enormous change in approach to regulation, and could be recommended only on a firm foundation of evidence.'[14] Meanwhile, attempts were being made by government via contract to persuade general practitioners to take part in continuing medical education by linking attendance at courses with their seniority payments for the NHS. There were no comparable professional arrangements at that time for specialists.

The main Merrison proposals were in relation to medical discipline and fitness to practice and of course the composition of the Council itself. In terms of the former, by far the biggest change was to recognise the problem of the sick doctor and to adopt the GMC's proposals for new machinery to deal with such cases. The establishment of the health procedures was important in a number of respects, not least that it required a different approach to the collection and analysis of evidence, and of the decisions to be made as a result. That decision was important. It certainly meant that professional colleagues felt more confident in referring doctors whose health was a possible risk to patients. Through this new sense of ownership they felt that the new system would be fair and supportive to doctors who were ill, rather than treating them as just another category of misconduct.

As to constitution, Merrison gave the profession what it had asked for at the cost of an enormously enlarged Council – an increase to 98

* Education Council for Foreign Medical Graduates.
† The American Board of Family Practice was the first of the American speciality boards to introduce periodic recertification in 1969.

members. I remember the discussions about fiddling with the numbers and the ultimate decision that the professionally elected majority should be decisive. But a caveat was added. To ensure that the educational function would not be compromised, the Education Committee was to be given independent statutory powers with a composition that would reflect its educational function.

Response to, and implementation of, Merrison

The profession was mightily relieved that, from its point of view, the constitutional issue had been resolved in favour of an unambiguous majority of doctors elected by the profession. But there was less agreement about some of the substantive proposals. Specialist registration clearly posed problems for the consultants. They appeared to feel that an 'accreditation' might be devised to satisfy the continental and therefore EEC inclusive view of what a specialist is, but not for the 'higher' British view of a consultant. But it was the reactions to graduate clinical training – the new pre-registration year – that I found most disappointing. I represented the RCGP at the GMC conference on the registration and educational implications of Merrison in July 1976. Speaker after speaker gave reasons only why change would be difficult.

Nevertheless, the GMC and the BMA were keen to get the proposals implemented, but it was not until November 1977 that a Bill was finally put before the Lords. The government originally accepted the Committee's recommendations for a reconstituted GMC, that the GMC should have responsibility for co-ordinating all stages of medical education and that it should maintain an indicative specialist register. It agreed in principle on the need to change the mode of registration of overseas-trained doctors; it also agreed that the GMC should be able to control the registration of doctors whose health endangered patients. These were significant improvements for both the profession and patients.

But in the event the government limited its proposals about medical education to undergraduate education; there was nothing about the registration of overseas-trained doctors or about giving the GMC powers to offer positive guidance on professional standards. It indicated that on these further discussion was needed. So the GMC and the BMA enlisted the help of John Hunt (by now Lord Hunt of Fawley), a past-President of the RCGP, to lead an assault on the Bill in the House of Lords. Hunt threw himself into the task with the GMC and the BMA, and succeeded in achieving a remarkable degree of agreement within the profession about the missing recommendations on postgraduate medical training, the maintenance of standards and the registration of overseas-trained doctors. Lord Wells-Pestell, spokesman for the Labour government in the Lords,[29] said:

> During the last month circumstances [about possible professional disagreements] have changed dramatically . . . and at an unprecedented speed. I have never known so much agreement to be achieved in so little time. The General Medical Council, the British Medical Association and the Overseas Doctors Association felt it so important that the Bill's provision should be extended to implement Merrison's recommendations on a variety of matters that an unexpected consensus has emerged on these matters amongst those groups as to which form the provisions should take.

As a result of this working together, the government effectively capitulated with good grace and amended the Bill in these respects, thus adding further to the sense of a great step forward.[5]

There is a rather ironic tailpiece. John Hunt was the effective founder of the College of General Practitioners. An outstanding general practitioner in private general practice, he moved in the highest medical circles in London and so knew all the grandees at the top of the profession. His own college – the Royal College of Physicians of London – had been supremely indifferent to the problems of standards in general practice. Nevertheless when Hunt proposed a new college to deal with this, the RCP strove vigorously to strangle the upstart college at birth. The President of the RCP refused to speak to Hunt for some time after the College of General Practitioners was founded.

Towards the end of his term as President of the College, the government offered John Hunt a CBE in recognition of his achievements. He and the close circle of colleagues he consulted thought this was an insult to general practice. He had after all rendered the public as well as general practice a major service in founding a college concerned primarily with standards of practice. However the feeling was that it just had to be accepted that, at that stage in the development of the speciality, a knighthood was beyond a general practitioner, however good they were and however great their contribution had been. The tribal influences reached right into the heart of government.

But Hunt was highly regarded by the parliamentary opposition. Very shortly afterwards he emerged as a Conservative life peer. We were all delighted. And here was the twist. If the Establishment had given him the knighthood he deserved originally, he would not have been in the House of Lords when the crunch came on Merrison. So the chances are that we would have had, as Stacey[5] put it, 'half a bill, practically worthless', because no one in the Lords at the time would have had either the ability or willingness to lead on this subject as effectively as he did.

The Merrison Report in retrospect

The Merrison Committee was a major learning experience for me. The membership, both lay and medical, was very strong. Merrison himself was a very clear thinker and Cecil Clothier, a barrister non-medical member, had a razor-sharp mind for regulatory matters. The Secretary to the Committee, Brian Bridges, was also a clear thinker and writer, as the report showed. I emerged from that experience with a great deal more knowledge and understanding than I had at the beginning. It confirmed in my mind the potential power of registration as a guarantor of doctors' professionalism. Merrison represented a big step forward in terms of enfranchising the whole of the profession and the subsequent enactment of the health proposals was to prove as beneficial as people had hoped. It still has relevance in today's climate. The proposals on specialist registration and the pre-registration year required a quantum shift in the cultural mindset of the universities and colleges, which at that stage they were not prepared to make. However, the discussions had begun and could not – and would not – be ignored.

From the patient's point of view the changes were limited and conservative. The whole exercise was very doctor/profession orientated, as by its terms of reference it was bound to be, reflecting the way society and the profession saw matters 25 years ago. The concept of the Medical Register as a list of the competent was as fundamental then as it is today – but only on joining the Register. Steps taken by a doctor subsequently to keep up to date were to continue to be voluntary and linked almost exclusively to continuing medical education.

The illumination of the GMC's and the government's approach to overseas-trained doctors provides one of the most important lessons for today. The consequences for patients of the regulator compromising its independence on standards to suit a health service looking for a quick fix of cheap labour were severe. By not tackling it effectively, too many patients were put at risk. Equally too many excellent doctors who trained outside the UK and EEC have been treated badly – too often exposed to poor training, then poor job choices in shortage specialities in under-privileged parts of the country. The Merrison response was only partial. The RCGP proposal, a proper entry test for all doctors entering the UK from any country, would I believe have assured the public of a uniform standard directly comparable to that demanded of UK graduates – one standard for registration. It would have been fair and non-discriminatory to all doctors trained outside the UK, putting them on a directly comparable basis with those graduating from UK medical schools.

It confirmed in my mind that employers – including the NHS – should never be allowed to become effectively the licensing body. The conflict of interest is just too strong. When the chips are down, when there is a real shortage of doctors, the temptation to 'dumb down' on standards can be understandably overpowering. We need to reflect on that today. We have an open door policy with Europe because there is free movement of doctors. What happens when the EEC is enlarged, to admit some countries which do not have medical training standards comparable to our own?

Perhaps the most interesting insights are about medical standards and the development of the relationship between the profession and the public. There had been demands from some for a code of practice to give doctors a better idea of what might lead them to be disciplined. But the Merrison Committee accepted the GMC's thinking that continuing to build on 'case law' as had been done historically was preferable. That policy did not change until the GMC introduced *Good Medical Practice* and linked that to registration, nearly 30 years later. The Committee did, however, strongly recommend that the GMC's advice in the *Blue Book* should be considerably expanded so that doctors would know better what constituted unacceptable behaviour.

The Alment Committee: competence to practise

The Alment Committee[30] followed hard on the heels of Merrison, and tried to deal with the issue that Merrison had set aside as being too difficult, namely 'the maintenance of standards of continuing competence to practise and of the clinical care of patients.' This Committee, instigated by the Board of Science of the BMA, was wholly professional, including mainly representatives of the Royal Medical Colleges and Faculties, the Joint Consultants' Committee and the BMA. Again I was involved, representing the RCGP.

At that time, it was known that various developments on the assessment of ongoing competence were taking place overseas, and medical audit was beginning to be developed in this country. The question was whether and how these, together with developments in continuing medical education, could contribute to assessing ongoing competence. All this was against the background of awareness that, certainly in the case of general practice but not really admitted in the consultant service, there were concerns about the competence of some doctors. Variation in standards had become steadily more stark in general practice as good practices moved ahead whilst others did not. I had already pinned my colours publicly to the mast. In 1975 I said in my RCGP William Pickles lecture:[24]

> The public has noticed. Complaints about badly run appointments' systems and principals who are habitually unavailable for emergency

care are too common for comfort: these contrast vividly with the praise given to well-run practices. When it comes to clinical standards the few public complaints are no consolation because lay people have difficulty in commenting objectively on technical matters. However, evidence is accumulating, especially from prescribing patterns, the College's membership examination and our clinical colleagues in hospital, of variations in the quality of the clinical practice of individual doctors, which is unacceptably wide . . . This variation points inexorably to our unwillingness to pursue systematically [a policy of agreeing] minimal clinical and operational standards for all doctors . . . We have been unable to offer the public a guarantee of minimum performance.

I concluded that in general practice we could no longer avoid the introduction of explicit professional standards as a requirement for every family doctor.

I remember the first meeting of the Alment Committee. The atmosphere was quite different from Merrison. Even on that first day, despite the best efforts of the Chairman, protective positions were already being taken up. In a sense it was doomed from the start. Alment himself was President of the Royal College of Obstetricians and Gynaecologists (RCOG). He was very much concerned with standards and had been responsible for quite major reforms to improve healthcare for women. He believed in professional standards and transparency, reflected in words I remember he often used to repeat: 'Let there be no hiding place.' Such transparency about clinical results was indicative of a man with a strong sense of social and professional responsibility, and far-sightedness.

The report, published in 1976, talked in general terms about re-certification and re-licensure. The value of taking part in medical audit was carefully explained and the work of professional enthusiasts was warmly encouraged and endorsed. However, throughout the emphasis was on a voluntary process in which standards were 'best determined by doctors in the course of actual care of their own patients'. From this it was deduced that there was as yet no evidence to justify re-licensure:[30]

. . . not because there is no evidence that doctors fail in their competence in certain respects and that this can be detected, but rather because a system of licensing for all could not be based upon measurements satisfactory enough to justify it . . . Such a system would impose a demand for conformity in a situation in which the public is best served by diversity. It would replace trust in individuals by trust in systems in the professional field where the trusted individual is the cornerstone of good practice.

One of the most prophetic statements was its recognition that 'in today's fast-moving society . . . a plea for protection from control mechanisms for a selected group of individuals who possess knowledge and skills of importance to the general public may well seem to be special pleading'. Quite so!

The report sank without trace, leaving no impact on the profession or government. The inquiry was regarded by some as a missed opportunity to get to grips with the growing problem of continuing competence and performance. In conversations I had at the time and subsequently with Alment, I know how disappointed he was that good intentions and high aspirations could so quickly fall in the light of the harsh realities of medical trade union power at the time. As a signatory to the report, I was part of the failure. My recollection is that the profession, as represented by the vast majority on the Committee, was simply not prepared to confront the problem seriously. At that time those, including myself, who wanted to do so were simply too weak or unskilled to force our views across. This episode together with Merrison's ducking of re-certification were significant, if understandable, failures of professional self-regulation.

6

Some spirits were willing but . . . , 1980–90

A new boy on the Council

I had been one of the many new members of the GMC in 1979. I was appointed by the RCGP, which had its own representative on the GMC for the first time. I had come to the GMC with no previous experience of it, but good recent knowledge of its work through my membership of the Merrison Inquiry.

As we new members found our feet, tribal behaviours were in evidence. For example, in the main university and college members preferred to concentrate on medical education matters and to leave the long and at times tedious business of sitting on conduct committee panels to elected members. The BMA, which had lobbied so strongly to get its own members elected, formed a discernible presence through many of its prominent Council members, and established its own informal lobby. The overseas-qualified doctors formed a distinctive, close-knit group. The lay members did not identify themselves overtly as a lobby, but rather maintained an independence of action that simply added to their effectiveness. But Ian Kennedy, who came on as a lay member in 1984, told me recently that there were informal conversations about the best tactics to use to try to get the GMC to tackle poor practice.

John Richardson was firm but fair as President. He made it clear that members were there to serve the GMC, and to do that they needed to leave their other professional hats at the door. For some this was impossible, but it was good to see how many did act as independent-minded representatives and not delegates.

I remember also how surprised I was that the GMC was so legalistic in its approach. Everything was related to the Medical Act, which was the statutory basis for its operations. This gave the impression – and indeed the reality – of a much narrower and inward-looking perspective on the medical profession and its regulation than I had perhaps come to expect from my wider experience outside. Part of the problem was institutional boundaries. The GMC was still heavily orientated around specialist medicine. So it was very deferential to the Colleges and at the same time wary of them. I soon discovered, for example, that the Colleges undermined discreetly any serious attempts by the GMC Education Committee to be effective in co-ordinating all stages of medical education. The GMC was beginning to get some good ideas, for example the Education Committee, led by Professor Arthur Crisp, produced excellent recommendations on specialist training in 1987.[31] But nothing happened. The combination of educational conservatism and territorial tribalism in the Colleges was too difficult to overcome. As the Colleges saw it these areas were their preserve. Whatever had been said by Merrison, the GMC was not expected to interfere.

The Council was big. As we were all to learn, it was a place where people came to make speeches, not least to be heard by their electorate. I found it quite intimidating. The format was not conducive to thoughtful policy development or to the exploration of ideas. Each February there was an informal internal conference that gave more of an opportunity to explore issues of the day, but they were one-off events and they did not create an environment that encouraged discussions or follow-through outside the conference.

An outstanding problem was the growing dissonance between a very doctor-oriented Council that, like the profession it represented, was reluctant to open the Pandora's box of poorly performing doctors, and the public, the press and some within the profession itself, who thought that it must. It is helpful to bear in mind that the BMA believed that it was dealing adequately with poor practice through the NHS complaints and employment arrangements. On the other hand consumer activists believed it was the GMC, not the BMA nor the NHS, that was there to protect them from poor practice.

In the 1970s and 1980s, people's attitudes to health and healthcare were changing as the consumer and patients' rights movements took a real hold in Britain, especially in respect of childbirth and maternity care. In medicine the march of scientific discovery and technological development continued apace with all that implied for the costs of healthcare. Doctors' attitudes to the concept of 24-hour personal service were changing as the row between general practice and the government over out-of-hours care and deputising showed. More women were coming into medicine and with that came the requirement for more flexible working, not always reconcilable with some long-established working practices in some specialities.

The 1980s also marked a turning point for the NHS, with the election of a Conservative government led by Margaret Thatcher. The growing consumer revolution began to impact on general health policy and therefore on the GMC. There was a belief at the time of her re-election in 1983 that Mrs Thatcher had no great aspirations to reform healthcare services, but rather that she grew tired of repeated criticisms of the NHS. The NHS itself lurched from one financial crisis to another. Earlier reorganisations, by both Labour and Conservative administrations, had merely shuffled the structural arrangements without affecting the mode of service delivery in any serious way at all. Under Kenneth Clarke's leadership, in 1989 there was the first of the major reforms called *Working for Patients*.

General practice had its own Waterloo. *The 1990 Contract* introduced more performance management to an 'independent contractor' service, and with it performance-related incentive payments. It was bitterly resented by the BMA and split the RCGP.

Kenneth Clarke provoked strong reactions. I remember him speaking at an RCGP dinner in 1989, when he made a joke about GPs 'feeling for their wallets' whenever quality was mentioned. Everyone was highly appreciative of the joke at the time – he was a very entertaining speaker – until it got out to the profession, when there was fury at what was perceived by some as an insult. However, the BMA had its own back. I remember the BMA advertisement – ' What do you call a man who does not take medical advice?' – with a picture of Clarke alongside. Clarke always said that the correct answer should be 'Healthy.'

The Thatcher reforms in healthcare were by far the most significant since the formation of the NHS itself. They were deeply opposed by the opposition parties and many in the medical profession. Most significantly from the politicians' point of view, they became unpopular with the general public.

Quality in general practice

As with the previous decade, there were four major developments in general practice. They are particularly relevant to the central theme of this book – medical culture and the development of medical professionalism.

In 1982 I was elected Chairman of the RCGP Council, and thus in a better position to do something about the unacceptably wide variation in the quality of general practice. This was still for patients the outstanding problem.[32] There had undoubtedly been huge improvements in much of general practice, but that only made the contrast between the best and the poorest even starker. It was all very well for the patients of good practices but hardly right for those who were not. And, as consumers' organisations pointed out, patients did not always have a choice of practice, particularly in inner cities and the bigger conurbations, or in some rural communities.

So I proposed to the RCGP Council that we as a College showed leadership on this matter. In what became known as *The RCGP Quality Initiative*,[33] we decided as a Council 'to change attitudes and habits in general practice', to change the culture by aiming to adopt 'standard setting and performance review as a normal part of a college member's way of life'. To give practical effect to this cultural change we said that each general practitioner should be able to describe their services to patients. Against that description, each doctor should then define specific care and health objectives for the care of patients and monitor the extent to which they were met. We set a target of ten years for implementation throughout the profession. In the event it was over-optimistic, but it was important that by setting ourselves a target we were modelling a rigorous approach.

Virtually the whole Council volunteered for the *Quality Initiative*. Very soon after, the faculties or local branches of the RCGP across the country became involved. Around the quarterly Council meetings, we set aside time for members to present their individual audits. We established a newsletter and fast communications system* so that members could share experiences, learn from each other, and support and encourage colleagues. Avedis Donabedian, then the leading international figure in conceptualising and assessing clinical quality in healthcare, accepted an invitation to come over from the USA to spend a month at the College. He visited most parts of the country and was a powerful stimulator and giver of practical advice. For me it was a great personal pleasure to learn at first hand from this wise man.

As part of the *Quality Initiative*, a small group of Council members started developing a grid of data indicative of four areas of a doctor's performance – professional values, accessibility, clinical competence and an ability to communicate. Known as *What Sort of Doctor?*[34] it sparked a new line of development of personal and practice review. This would find its ultimate expression in the RCGP *Fellowship by Assessment* (FBA), a very robust and sophisticated approach to reviewing the performance of an established general practitioner. FBA was the inspiration and brainchild of Denis Pereira Gray, another outstanding leader who had a general practice known widely for its quality of patient care.

---

* Edited by the late Bill Styles, the Honorary Secretary, and Sally Fountain (now Irvine), the General Administrator.

At the same time, as another part of the *Quality Initiative*, the then Honorary Secretary of the College, John Hasler, and the late Nancy Dennis (a lay person) established the Patients' Liaison Group, to bring the patients' perspective of quality right into the heart of the College. This was the first time a medical Royal College had brought patients directly into its affairs. We also attempted unsuccessfully to broaden the base of the College to include other clinical and non-clinical members of the practice team, in the belief that the pursuit of quality had to become a team-based enterprise. But that was a bridge too far, and the Council and I were soundly rebutted by the College members at the Spring General Meeting in 1984 when we tried to take this through.

In turn the interest in quality generated much interest in audit, using the principles of the *Quality Initiative*. In my own region general practitioners, paediatricians and health service researchers carried out the first national major multi-practice study of standard setting and performance assessment in general practice.[35] The trainers constructed working clinical guidelines for five common conditions of childhood, which together gave a representative picture of general practitioners' performance. Data on performance were abstracted from the clinical records before and after the standard-setting activities, and then compared. The effects of giving performance feedback were studied. The process and outcome study was able to demonstrate significant changes in some clinical outcomes.* [36,37]

The problem with all these developments in general practice was that they were voluntary. Uptake was quite limited. That did not help patients who wanted consistency of care for all across all parts of the medical profession. As far as general practice was concerned the government wanted to give general practitioners incentive payments – known as the *Good Practice Allowance* – for being involved in the quality improvement activities on which the College was leading. The BMA declined. So in the 1990 Contract the government imposed its own ideas about a performance-related contract. The BMA's position was founded on its apparently unshakeable belief that progress could only be made at the speed set by the conservative majority that did not want performance-related incentives – a not unreasonable position for a representative body to take. In summary therefore whilst there was a lot of good practice, there was at the same time an unwillingness on the part of the BMA to get to grips with poor practice.

---

* In fact several of today's national experts on clinical guidelines, such as Allen Hutchinson, Martin Eccles and Jeremy Grimshaw, cut their teeth in this study.

The patients' revolt

It was precisely this kind of situation that led to what Margaret Stacey has referred to as 'the era of the patients' revolt'.[5] Important voices, albeit few in number, were beginning to be raised about the GMC's effectiveness in dealing with poor practice. One of the most articulate and influential expressions of the consumer views of the medical profession and its regulator was given voice by Professor Ian Kennedy. Kennedy was a trenchant critic of medical practice as it was then. In his prescient Reith lectures, published in 1981 under the title of *The Unmasking of Medicine*,[38] he doubted whether the self-regulation of doctors would be adequate at the end of the 20th century. He argued that while the GMC had a primary duty to protect the public interest, it had no efficient mechanism for asking the public what that interest was. Indeed too many complaints were dismissed without lay involvement and without open examination and public scrutiny. It was not effectively held to account by the Privy Council. He was concerned at the extent to which the GMC's disciplinary role (what complaints it should deal with) was 'resource led' – that is, determined by the amount of money the GMC was prepared to spend on investigating and hearing cases.

Kennedy's solution was a much more proactive GMC that would insist on regular re-registration (now called revalidation). It would include some sort of inspectorate able to look at any aspect of professional practice, including issues like communication with patients and ethics. However, this would need specific guidelines as to what constituted good practice.

Jean Robinson, who had a wide knowledge of patients' complaints through her work for the Patients' Association, represented consumers as a lay member. She was another important and courageous critic within the Council itself. She had an assertive style that many GMC members, particularly the male professionals, found uncomfortable. This was not surprising as she was frequently touching sensitive nerves when she confronted the Council with the inadequacy of its policies on poor clinical practice when seen from the viewpoint of the public rather than the medical profession. In 1988 she published a devastating critique of the Council's performance in the 1980s,[39] highlighting its lack of transparency and its unwillingness to grasp the issue of professional competence properly.

But the real power of her contribution came in the GMC meetings themselves because Council meetings were held in public and members had to face up to the consumer perspective that she championed. Some medical members demonised her – I thought wrongly – for putting her views and those of the consumers she represented so assertively and directly. Her testimony is the more powerful because of whom she was addressing and the circumstances.

Rudolph Klein, then Professor of Social Policy at the University of Bath, focused on issues of doctors' accountability.[40] 'Once a doctor has graduated onto the medical register', he noted, 'the GMC's role is essentially negative.' It reacts to complaints, particularly about doctors' personal conduct. 'It does not deal with the doctor who is neither psychiatrically ill nor dishonest, who does not touch drink or drugs, who does not sleep with his patients or break the law, but has simply lost interest in his profession: who is a good and sane citizen but a poor doctor.' The GMC saw its role, he asserted, as to 'drum convicted sinners out of the profession, not to ensure continued professional virtue'.

Margaret Stacey was a lay member of the GMC between 1976 and 1984. She subsequently embarked on a sociological analysis of the Council for the same period, which I have cited already, to put flesh on the bones of her experience. It is the most authoritative descriptive audit of the work of the GMC that exists.[5] Its great value is that it was written through the eyes and ears of a member of the public who believed in the principle of self-regulation but who was refreshingly unsentimental about what was needed to make it work properly for patients.

Her preference was for self-reform. She held that any labour force works better if its members have some sense of ownership for the regulator under which they work. Regulation from above or outside she felt could lead to the alienation of those being regulated.

But external critics of the GMC also came from the profession. The editor of the *BMJ*, Stephen Lock, had asked his editorial assistant, Richard Smith, to research several sensitive subjects, including the GMC, health centres, the prison medical services and product liability. Smith went exhaustively into the workings of the Council and spoke widely with people, lay and medical. In the summer of 1989 the *BMJ* published a series of nine papers profiling the GMC. These papers were offered in a spirit of constructive criticism. Perhaps indicative of his own feelings, Smith described the GMC as 'a nineteenth century institution trying – and largely failing – to adapt to the late twentieth century'. 'The day of judgement comes closer' he wrote, as for some at least the GMC was seen as 'progressively losing touch with a fast-changing world'.[41]

Smith's critique was devastating for the GMC because it came from an influential and respected doctor. Lock, in a subsequent editorial in the *BMJ*,[42] summarised Smith's main conclusions. The GMC was too large and its powers were too concentrated in its subcommittees. Despite over half the members being elected, there were too few young doctors and too many academics. Internal problems seemed to preoccupy members and staff more than, for example, the need for better supervision in education and the issues of clinical incompetence. Lastly he wrote that the Council had to be seen to be serving the public interest. It should not, as it seemed to do, resent the 'unfairness' of pressure by the media or by MPs representing anxious or dissatisfied constituents.

Lock, clearly with Smith's agreement, wanted an independent inquiry to deal with the major issues raised by Smith's articles. Such an inquiry, he urged, should not neglect the power of the GMC secretariat, headed by the registrar. Although uncertain as to how much power resided there, Smith and Lock had concluded that the permanent staff were 'likely to set the prevailing tone that operates – in particular poor communications, both internally and externally'.

Kennedy's Reith lectures were a wake-up call from the public, but there were doctors who were pretty critical of his thesis. Jean Robinson's efforts were applauded in the consumer world, and certainly got through to ministers, whilst being disregarded by doctors. Rudolf Klein sustained his arguments for properly accountable professional practice and regulation. Stacey's book was I thought fair but to the point – she told me later that some senior medical people on the GMC and in the secretariat tried to stop her publishing it in the form she intended. She prepared for legal action because she was not prepared to modify her findings. However, in the event it was not necessary.

But it was the Smith papers that evoked most reaction, particularly in the GMC. The President, Robert Kilpatrick, published a response article[43] in the *BMJ* under the title 'Profiles of the GMC: portrait or caricature?' In responding to some of the more important criticisms, he observed that Richard Smith had offered little by way of hard evidence to support many of his adverse comments. Nor had he attempted to balance the comments of well-known GMC critics with views from those who thought otherwise just as sincerely. Kilpatrick wrote, 'I must say that what I have seen of the GMC's work in my 13 years service bears little resemblance to the body described in Dr Smith's profile.' Behind the scenes, Robert Kilpatrick and several other very senior members made their complaints known to one of the regular officer meetings of the BMA – although the *BMJ* is editorially independent of the BMA. But some of us felt uncomfortable about the defensive reactions for in truth there was much that was true, and needed attention.

Margaret Stacey's book was not published until 1992. However, I regret very much that we did not have a proper discussion in the Council in the 1980s of the critiques by Smith, Robinson, Kennedy and Klein. We should have confronted the issues head on. As the Chairman of the Standards Committee from 1984, I should – and probably could – have done more, at least to get a debate going. It was one of those 'if only' moments, which one lives to regret.

Confronting clinical incompetence

So what actually was the GMC doing both in the face of the competence issues in general practice which were known about widely, and the growing criticism of its perceived lack of interest in the subject? I have given some space here to describe the Council's discussions in public at Council meetings, in order to give a feel for the mood, the arguments and the tensions. The 1980s began with the GMC on the defensive, and concluded with a decision to develop a new methodology and set of fitness-to-practice procedures to deal specifically with poor clinical performance – and it was quite a journey.

Alfie Winn

The case of Alfie Winn, a young boy from Sheffield who had died of meningitis in 1982, stands out as the defining moment when the GMC first began to acknowledge that it had to take some responsibility for incompetent practice. Alfie was registered with Dr Arthur Archer, his general practitioner. In 1982 he became ill with vomiting and high temperature. The doctor was called. Dr Archer came three hours later. He asked the boy to open his mouth. The boy seemed comatose and his mother said, 'He can't hear you.' Dr Archer said, 'If he can't be bothered to open his bloody mouth, I shall not bloody well look at him.' He prescribed an antibiotic. Two hours later the family called an ambulance and Alfie was taken to hospital. Four days later he died. In March 1983 the GMC Professional Conduct Committee (PCC) heard the case. In the determination they were 'disturbed' by the failure to arrange specialist care and by the 'poor standard of courtesy' shown to Alfie's parents. The Committee regarded such behaviour as 'below the standard that can be regarded as acceptable in a medical man.' Nevertheless, taking account of Archer's expressions of regret they considered that there was no serious professional misconduct.

Nigel Spearing, Mrs Winn's MP, wrote to the GMC in June 1983. In the light of the Committee's decision that he found completely unsatisfactory, he proposed that the GMC's powers should be strengthened by the removal of the word 'serious' from the charge of serious professional misconduct. The GMC set up a working group to consider the validity of Mr Spearing's proposal, in particular for the Preliminary Proceedings Committee (PPC) and PCC, in reaching their determinations. It reported in 1984 and concluded that it could find no evidence to justify lowering the threshold of SPM.[44] However, it did say that it would be helpful and beneficial to the public if there were detailed guidance on the circumstances in which failure to provide a sufficient standard of medical care might give rise to a case of SPM. This was all very tentative. The report also recommended that the PCC should give brief reasons for their decisions, which it had not previously done.

The Council considered the report from the Standards Committee on Friday 2 November 1984, the outline of which had been drafted by the then President, Sir John (later Lord) Walton. It approved a statement that the public was entitled to expect that a registered medical practitioner would afford and maintain a good standard of medical care. The statement, quite short, was nevertheless explicit in dealing with the essentials of good clinical care. It was the first time that the GMC had set out a statement of good clinical practice with such clarity. John Walton's initiative represented an important step forward and became one of the cornerstones of the GMC's *Good Medical Practice*, published some ten years later.

The Council debate[45] on the statement and report really gave a flavour of the anxieties, and the widely differing opinions held by members on the issue of competence. Jean Robinson went to the nub of the differences in attitude and expectation between the public and their doctors. She said:

> Mr President, I am very well aware that this is a most delicate subject for doctors to discuss and one could hardly be a member of this body for any length of time without realising how very vulnerable the members of the profession feel, when we as outsiders see them as almost invulnerable. So there is a great difference between us.

She welcomed the very clear definition of what the Council expected in the way of quality and style of medical care from the profession. She thought the statement was something that ordinary people could understand and she hoped it would be widely publicised. However, she extended her definition of good care to include a sympathetic manner and courteous behaviour to patients. She assured the Council, once again, that the public did not want to hammer any doctor who made an ordinary mistake in the course of a good professional life. Nevertheless the public did look to the Council to make sure that, by and large, doctors were practising a reasonable standard of medical care. She believed that the GMC still wanted to duck the main issue, that is, of allowing more complaints, particularly clinical complaints, to be fully investigated.

The issue of competence would not go away. In January 1985, the President met the Lord President of the Privy Council and the Chief Medical Officer of England (CMO) to discuss a consultation document from the GMC outlining proposed revisions to the way in which a doctor's fitness to practice was handled. However, the Privy Council and the health departments were proposing to change the law along the lines indicated by Spearing. The Council opposed this successfully.

In September 1986 Michael O'Donnell, a well-known medical member of Council, wrote an article for *BMA News Review* entitled 'A raw deal for all'.[46] In this article he concluded that the Professional Conduct Committee was an inappropriate mechanism for dealing with cases of alleged incompetence. His preference was for some alternative to the adversarial approach in current use, especially when issues of lapses in a doctor's skill or judgement were concerned. He described the rising sense of unease – shared by many of us serving on professional conduct committees – that, whilst specific allegations might not be proved to the criminal standard, nevertheless we were looking at evidence of a poor standard of practice. We were also seeing cases after considerable delay in investigation. I reflected more than once, as a doctor was struck off for clinical misconduct, on the possible damage that might have been done between the case first being reported and action finally being taken by the PCC itself.

In May 1987, due to increasing criticism of the Council's disciplinary procedures from within the Council, Members of Parliament and others, Sir John asked the Council to appoint a working party:

> To review the procedures of the Council in relation to disciplinary cases in which it is alleged that a doctor has seriously neglected or disregarded his professional responsibilities to patients, and to report.

Mrs Robinson's response to Sir John's initiative in this provided the grit.[47]

> Mr President, you said that the figures indicate that the Council is taking a sterner line but I would suggest that this is not what the figures indicate. What they actually indicate is that a far smaller percentage of doctors are being found guilty of serious professional misconduct than before. This suggests that the working party should be supplied with more detailed statistics over a longer period of time so that people can see what the trend is, particularly in relation to the number of registered medical practitioners, because my research suggests that fewer doctors are being struck off the register than ever before; but I could be wrong and my figures are not yet detailed enough.

She was most articulate in putting the consumer's view. And of course her pointed questioning, for example about numbers, simply showed up the lack of data that the Council had – or rather did not have – to clarify her statements.

The working party reported to the Council in full in May 1989, under the new President, Sir Robert Kilpatrick. It recommended that:

1 The Council should now give further consideration to the issue of the establishment of competence procedures, and that such consideration

should include an evaluation of current and proposed arrangements for medical audit within the NHS. They should also take account of the position of doctors not practising in the NHS, who might not be subject to medical audit.

2 Proposals for such competence procedures should be formulated as a basis for discussion with the profession and other bodies.

3 The definition of serious professional misconduct should not be changed.

4 Minor alterations should be made to the conduct procedures and screening, including the involvement of a lay screener.

In the May Council debate many speakers were congratulatory. For example, Sir Herbert Duthie, a medical Council member, referred to it as 'a quiet revolution that is taking place'.

Others followed in a similar vein. Dr Anne Gruneberg, an elected medical member, gave an interesting historical comment. She said that when she first joined the Council in 1979, the Standards Committee had asked her to produce a paper on what she thought the role of the Council should be as far as enforcing standards was concerned. Her paper had concluded by saying 'until this Council addresses the problem of the incompetent doctor, it will not be carrying out the wishes of the public of this country'. The then President, Lord Richardson, had moved past her paper without comment. She told the Council that he had told her later that, as she put it, 'he was fully seized of the need for such consideration to be given but he found that the difficulties of it were overwhelming'. Anne concluded by hoping that the President and the GMC would not now be similarly overwhelmed by these difficulties.

However, Sir Michael Drury, then immediate past President of the RCGP, said what many felt. He was disappointed in the paper, not because of what it said, but because he did not feel that it was 'imbued with the sense of urgency and the importance that this topic deserved'. He hoped that the GMC would 'proceed with great rapidity', and inform the profession and the public quite clearly what the GMC was doing and how it was setting about it.

Jean Robinson was of a similar mind, welcoming the Council's 'eventual' move towards looking not just at the misconduct that a doctor may commit but at the questions of competence. But she felt that the paper expressed its intentions tentatively and not with the degree of urgency that the public would see to be necessary. Then she struck with more telling points. She referred to the weaknesses of local medical audit and related this to the enormous variations in the variability and quality of care across the country. She concluded that to look at audit and competence solely on the basis of 'local boys being in charge' was not acceptable from a lay point of view. Her point was that reliance on the

NHS to deal with poor practice was insufficient. The GMC always tried to get the NHS to deal with things first and see itself only as a point of reference of last resort.

But her stinging remarks went to the issue of serious professional misconduct and, for her, the fact that the Council appeared hardly to have moved at all. She concluded thus:

> The fact remains, after all the anxieties expressed in Parliament and after all the private members' bills and after all the concerns . . . . Yes, we have moved a bit on competence, not before time, but on this question of serious professional misconduct, the primary issue, we have not budged at all. We, sitting on the Professional Conduct Committee, shall be unable – not unwilling – to deal with doctors who we know are not safe to practice. That is a fact. I think it is unsatisfactory that that position should continue.

There was an explosive reaction, not least from the President who was clearly very irritated.

Finally, Sheila Adam, a young public health doctor who later became deputy CMO in England, emphasised the measure of agreement there was on what needed to be done. She linked some of the debate with wider considerations of medical paternalism. She said, 'The Council has to assure itself that all doctors are involved in regular, systematic peer review, and also assure itself that there are procedures to recognise and deal with problems in performance.'

But, for all the rhetoric and the urgings of people like Michael Drury, it was another full year – May 1990 – before the Council finally decided to establish a working party to 'consider arrangements for the identification and handling of serious deficiency in a doctor's professional performance and to make recommendations'.

In my own contributions to that debate I raised a number of tricky issues. I sought to clarify the difference between 'competence' and 'performance' as we had done at the RCGP.* I strongly favoured assessments of performance because they were much closer to real practice. I referred to the separate question of how the profession would combine the educational aspects of audit or performance review with the professional, regulatory aspects that the Council was now considering. I also raised the question of the local machinery that would be needed to make the new set-up work and how this would be reconciled with the central machinery through the GMC. This issue of the

---

* In the RCGP's terms, competence describes knowledge and skills. Performance describes what the doctor does within actual practice. In these terms a doctor can be competent but not necessarily – or always – perform well, but a doctor who is incompetent can never perform well.

adequacy of the local arrangements for handling and managing poorly performing doctors was to return with a vengeance when we came to the high-profile cases of the 1990s.

I referred to 'the very thorny question' of what the relationship would be between the professions' machinery locally and nationally on the one hand, and what the National Health Service management, through contract and other arrangements, would do on the other. For the NHS, I noted, would have a very strong interest in its own right in the performance of doctors. Lastly, I drew attention to the importance of patients' perceptions of performance that included not just knowledge and skill but personal qualities such as kindness – does the doctor come on time, will she listen, does she care? I suggested that the means of bringing a judgement or 'appraisal' of these qualities would be needed, acknowledging that it did not exist at that time.

There's one final postscript to this saga. Secretary of State Kenneth Clarke visited the GMC. I was one of the people present when he made it absolutely clear, without emotion, that the GMC had got to grip the question of the incompetent doctor and grip it soon. If it failed to do so he would act himself through Parliament.

The detail of this story is important because the received wisdom today is that the GMC's decision to go with what was to become the performance procedures in the 1990s was as a result of strongly proactive action. It was not. Such action had to be dragged out of the Council, as many of the medical members glanced over their shoulders, perhaps quite understandably, at what their colleagues might say in other places such as the craft committees of the BMA.

Rounding up the 1980s

Over this ten years I had came to understand the operational realities of the GMC better, and to appreciate the limits as well as the achievements of Merrison. In 1988 I wrote formally to the GMC thus:

1 The medical profession as a whole has a responsibility to see that young doctors receive an appropriate training for their speciality. The satisfactory completion of this training should be marked in future by an indicative specialist register (to include general practice) maintained by the GMC, on the basis of standards and assessments determined by the appropriate Royal Colleges.

2 The medical profession as a whole should now assume responsibility for ensuring that all practitioners maintain their knowledge and skills and so continue to reflect the principles of good practice throughout their working careers. The Royal Colleges and Faculties should be

asked to consider how their collegiate members/fellows could make this personal commitment through involvement in its standard setting and performance review activities.

3   Breaches in terms of service should be dealt with by a practitioner's contracting or employing authority. Wilfully sustained poor performance should continue to be dealt with by the GMC under the general heading of serious professional misconduct. Shabby clinical practice, that grey area falling between acceptable and persistently unacceptable behaviour, is not covered at present and should be. I favour machinery operated by the profession itself, using local professional mechanisms somewhat akin to those of doctors handling sick doctors.

4   Looking ahead, when standard setting and performance review have become more general, I believe that the profession should consider either voluntary re-licensure or face the possibility of required re-licensure through periodic appraisal for the specialist register.

5   Overall, the most constructive contribution which the medical profession could make at this time of upheaval in our healthcare system would be to grasp the nettle of quality assurance as a fact of every doctor's daily life. Both the public and the government would be mightily relieved if the profession would do this job itself as I believe it should.'

As with the RCGP *Quality Initiative* in 1982, I believed that every doctor needed to sign up to quality standards and quality monitoring as a fundamental part of modern professionalism. Then there could be no argument about the baseline of good practice, and there would be a secure and reliable starting point for identifying and dealing with outliers, a few of whom would be problem doctors. The principles of linking professional standards to registration and to include quality assurance within clinical teams were firmly established in my mind. This conceptualisation of standards-driven professionalism became the central thrust of my agenda as President, seven years later.

Margaret Stacey, Ian Kennedy, Richard Smith, Jean Robinson, Rudolph Klein and other key lay observers all came to the same conclusion. In the 1980s the new GMC was not functioning well, particularly with regard to its primary purpose of protecting the public. Stacey summed it up:[5]

It [the GMC] has not yet succeeded in renegotiating the education and training of doctors to the conditions of medicine of the late 20th century. It has never really ensured the continuing competence of registered practitioners.

All the evidence suggested that when she served on the Council in the decade in question, 'the Council had on balance resolved the many tensions it faced in regulating the profession in favour of the profession rather than the public'.

On the other hand Jean Robinson, when considering what hope there was for reform, concluded thus:[39]

> No medical profession in the developed world could have had a body of patients who are more docile and grateful than the British since the formation of the Health Service . . . Only when a sufficiently large number of patients and their relatives had been radicalised did we begin to see change, and a serious discussion of problems in the media . . . In the end consumer organisations did not have to work hard to convince the public that something was wrong – the doctors and their representatives were doing the job for them. How can doctors, most of whom are intelligent and kind, collectively be so dim?
>
> It seems to me that it is the very strength of the defences the medical profession has built around them that have prevented constructive change. The highly paid, high-powered defence lawyers, the skilful drafting of rules and regulations, the power of the profession in getting the kind of medical act and NHS complaint system they wanted, have prevented the emergence of underlying truth and constructive action. In the short term the doctors' organisations have been highly successful, but I believe that the long-term consequences have been damaging to individual doctors and to the profession as a whole.

So that was an alternative epitaph on the GMC in the 1980s.

But more optimistically I saw, with Stacey, that the Council at the outset of the 1990s was starting seriously to attempt to deal with continuing competence to practice and to address the other matters crucial to gaining both public and professional confidence. The real question, as Stacey said,[5] was whether it could go far enough. Would it be able to bring the BMA and the Royal Colleges with it? Would it be able to do that fast enough? Would the BMA and the Colleges, as well as the GMC, 'be able to stomach what is really needed – a reform of the Council which would change it beyond recognition, in which a great deal of the present power . . . would have to be ceded to others, in which among other things the lay voice was not only heard but understood and in which the Council's work was clearly articulated to the other bodies concerned with medical regulation'? Prophetic words indeed in the light of what was to happen.

7

Taking the initiative but losing the plot

The GMC in the early 1990s, optimistically, was working on several new emerging policies. But as we saw in the last chapter there was still a huge question mark over whether, as Stacey wondered, it would have the will and capacity for the radical reforms needed to modernise professional regulation.

We need however to put these issues into the perspective of the time. There were huge changes taking place both in the direction and the organisation of the NHS. At the same time British medicine was awakening to the revolution in the USA on the assessment of quality of healthcare. Compared with these the issues of professionalism, doctor's performance and medical regulation were low key and virtually subliminal. What the GMC was doing or not doing still went largely unnoticed on the wider national scene.

Working for patients

For people working in the NHS, the dominant factor of the early nineties was the impact of the Conservative government's NHS reforms. The Conservative plans had a powerful focus on consumer rights, quality of care and cost containment, and consequently had a strong transatlantic feel. The new legislation, based on the White Paper *Working for Patients*,[48] set the tone in earnest in 1990. It made explicit, as the title suggests, that the patient and not producer interests would be the primary focus of the NHS in the future. It attempted to bring commercial values to patient care and so improve quality through an internal market. In particular, it gave power to general practice through the fundholding experiment to act as an arbiter of quality on behalf of patients through the control of hospital budgets, and it enabled hospitals and community trusts to apply for self-governing status. Hierarchical NHS management was to be replaced by more local responsibility with decisions devolved to create competition and choice as stimulants to quality.

The medical political climate, particularly in general practice, was sharply divided on these reforms. Virtually the whole of specialist medicine was deeply against, mainly because it meant loss of direct control by specialists over their hospital budgets.

Fundholding in general practices was highly innovatory and, for some, provocative. Volunteer practices were to be given a budget from which they would provide most of their own services and purchase most care for their patients. Fundholding was bitterly opposed by a majority of GPs. Some were opposed to any change, or objected to the extra work they thought it would mean for them. Others – excellent practices – were ideologically opposed to a measure that they thought would damage the equity principle, by giving the patients of fundholders unfair advantage, particularly in access to secondary care. Some excellent small practices did not have the critical mass of patients required to hold a fund and so were ineligible.

Under the stimulus of *Working for Patients* the quality movement that was already stirring in parts of medicine made further progress. It was still seen in the medical community as a minority pursuit, one for 'anoraks'. However the adoption of the idea of evidence-based medicine in this country, the development of clinical guidelines and methods for assessing quality, and the rising volume of clinical auditing activities since the government had made audit a contractual requirement in the NHS were starting to change the medical culture. Such enthusiasm as there was for audit amongst clinicians generally was tempered by their quite specific requirement that it be professionally led, educational, formative, confidential, carried out only by peers and not directly linked to management processes. NHS trusts made clinical audit arrangements in their hospitals, and Medical Audit Advisory Groups (MAAGs) were established for general practitioners.[49] All doctors were encouraged and expected to take part.

There were other manifestations of this change. For example, the medical Royal Colleges began to introduce a professional requirement for doctors to undertake prescribed amounts of continuing medical education (known as Continuing Professional Development (CPD)). General practitioners were already contractually bound to CPD through the Postgraduate Education Allowance (PGEA) scheme, which linked a certain volume and quality of CPD involvement to their NHS income.

In 1993, the new CMO, Kenneth Calman, published a landmark report on specialist training.[50] The starting point was the need to harmonise specialist training in the UK with specialist training in the European Community. UK training was longer. His report recommended reducing the minimum length of specialist training to seven years. A new training grade of specialist registrar was created. These new proposals were tied up with alterations in junior doctors' hours. So effectively the state was drawn further into the traditionally professional area of training, not least because of the need to reconcile training with manpower requirements and career structures in the NHS. But there was a determination to improve the quality and supervision of early specialist training which many of us considered unsatisfactory, especially when compared with the well-structured, professionally delivered training which then existed in general practice. An important outcome, in 1995, was the establishment of the STA to oversee training, and to issue Certificates of Completion of Specialist Training (CCSTs).

Political fallout

The political fallout from *Working for Patients* was both serious and significant, and it was aggravated by the capacity problem. In the half decade to 1995, the NHS was becoming progressively more stretched, and clinicians were feeling much more pressure as a result of the internal market, management requirements and so on. It was becoming increasingly difficult to sustain morale against reforms that were unpopular, and quality developments that were seen by many health professionals as marginal to everyday practice. With notable exceptions in both the hospital service and general practice, opposition to the reforms from the medical profession was widespread and determined, effectively orchestrated by the BMA. Other health unions felt similarly threatened. The protest embraced the opposition political parties under the ideological charge of creeping privatisation. But privatisation, as Kenneth Clarke was always at pains to point out, was not for him the point of the exercise, although some of his ministerial and cabinet colleagues gave the clear impression it was. On the contrary he was, he claimed, intent on modernising the NHS by improving access to care, the quality and efficiency of service delivery and the quality of clinical outcomes.

So, overall, the medical profession was not taking kindly to government attempts to introduce more accountability. As the internal market focus slipped from quality to cost containment, it led to the Wildean jibe that the government knew 'the price of everything and the value of nothing'.*

So this was the backdrop to the beginning of positive changes in the GMC.

---

* Adapted from Oscar Wilde (1892) *Lady Windermere's Fan*, Act 3.

Getting some things right

In this period of huge political dynamism, the GMC seemed an odd mixture – like the curate's egg, good in parts. It was still old-fashioned, conservative and slow, with no overall policy framework, but there were some significant developments that justified the cautious optimism that I reflected at the end of the previous chapter. These involved an increase in the lay membership of the Council, the first attempt at regular collaboration with another health regulator, the United Kingdom Council for Nursing, Midwifery and Health Visiting (UKCC), and new approaches to the training of medical students, professional standards and the assessment of poorly performing doctors.

The voice of the public

Crucial to public confidence was the decision, implemented on 1 November 1996, to double the proportion of lay members on the Council (to 25 out of 104). The Privy Council appointed lay members to the GMC quite independently. Lay members had shown how they could influence the Council's policies despite their relatively small numbers. However, given those limited numbers, it required a great deal of courage and fortitude to make points, especially when they were developing lines of thinking which the majority of doctor members found uncomfortable.

In the early 1990s in spite of this discomfort, a positive feeling had been growing amongst medical members that the non-medical, patient or lay perspective was important in its own right, distinctively different from the doctor's view, and had to become part of the GMC's internal thinking. The patient's perspective on quality was clearly different from that of the doctor. Even when the messages were uncomfortable, most doctors could see that a proper understanding of the public and patients' perspective was vital.

At the same time there was growing outside pressure for change, though still at that stage not a significant force. There was a growing feeling in and around Parliament that the public should have a bigger stake, and there were some MPs who wanted self-regulation to be replaced by a council with a lay majority. The push for greater public involvement was not confined to the GMC. The government intended far more public involvement in the NHS as part of its repositioning around the patient, hence for example *The Citizens' Charter*.

Working with nurses

Today there is much emphasis, rightly, on co-operative working between the regulators of the health professions. This process started in the early nineties between the GMC and the UKCC. The initiative came from the nurses. I was a member of both bodies at the time, and helped to get this started. Meetings in which we shared information and thinking continued right through my presidency.

Tomorrow's Doctors

A highly significant development involved the training of medical students. The Education Committee is responsible for the purpose and broad content of the undergraduate medical curriculum, and for the pre-registration year, the first year of being a doctor immediately after initial qualification. In practice this means that students follow detailed curricula devised by individual medical schools within the guidelines set by the GMC's Education Committee. Similarly in the first year of practice – the pre-registration year – the new doctor has to be supervised in posts that conform to GMC guidelines. Historically students spent their first two years gaining a sound knowledge of anatomy and physiology before being introduced to patients and their illnesses in the three remaining years. That is the system in which I trained.

Since the Second World War there had been a huge expansion in the knowledge base and in the complexity of medicine, which led to progressive specialisation, including general practice. It was clear that the predominantly knowledge-based course was becoming increasingly burdensome to medical students. Medical training was becoming a test of memory rather than the basis for real learning. Equally the reality of specialist training, particularly the adoption of mandatory training for general practice in 1982, produced a new opportunity to reconstruct the basic curriculum and give it new purpose and direction.

Some medical schools – Newcastle was the earliest example – had already started experimenting with a different approach to give students a broad experience of medicine on which postgraduate training could then build. They adopted a new curriculum, in which students were introduced to patients from the very beginning of their medical course. The new medical schools, Southampton, Nottingham and Leicester for example, designed their courses around the new thinking. Such innovations were popular with students and teachers. They were usually combined with new teaching methods that incorporated learning in small groups and a much greater use of continuous assessment. However, as the GMC Education Committee noted, in the majority of universities the perception of what newly qualified doctors should know and be capable of doing had not altered significantly in the eyes of either their teacher and examiners or of those for whom they would work as house officers.

So in the early 1990s, under the chairmanship of Professor David Shaw who was Dean of Medicine at Newcastle University, the Education Committee returned to the task with a new sense of determination. The result was *Tomorrow's Doctors*,[51] a radical blueprint for the future. In his introduction, David Shaw revealed the Education Committee's frustration with past inertia when he said, 'Notwithstanding repeated exhortation, there remains gross overcrowding of most undergraduate curricula, acknowledged by teachers and deplored by students. The scarcely tolerable burden of information that is imposed taxes the memory but not the intellect.' Why the inertia? Because the medical schools (like individual doctors) had a highly developed sense of autonomy and they were not going to be told what to do by anybody, including the GMC that regulated them. It was in the culture, and past experience had taught them that non-compliance did not lead to sanction.

So *Tomorrow's Doctors* presented the medical schools with an opportunity and with a challenge. There was the opportunity within the new framework for real experiment and innovation if medical schools were prepared to show leadership. But there was an expectation that this time the basic framework must be implemented. Through a programme of inspection visits to the medical schools, the Education Committee would check on compliance and seek explanation and reasons where there were significant departures. That power had always existed but hitherto the Committee had chosen not to use it. In serious cases it could recommend to the Privy Council that recognition be withdrawn.

The foundation of *Tomorrow's Doctors* was a core curriculum that set out in modern terms what the medical student should be able to master by the time of qualification. The ethos was student-centred learning with more emphasis on the quality of teaching. Essentially, the committee wanted to give the universities a very clear steer as to what was expected in terms of the 'core' whilst leaving ample scope for individual medical schools to innovate and experiment through a series of supplementary special study modules. These modules gave students opportunities to explore particular interests in medicine, in healthcare generally or even outside the health system altogether.

Tomorrow's Doctors was more patient-oriented than the old curricula. In addition to early exposure to patients, there was far more emphasis on the development of interpersonal skills, particularly of communication skills. Public health medicine and general practice were to become required contributors to the curriculum. Overall it involved a serious change in the educational culture of medicine.

The medical schools took up *Tomorrow's Doctors* with varying degrees of enthusiasm. David Shaw and his team spent much time visiting their colleagues in medical schools to work through the new approach and to encourage them to take ownership. The CMO helped by making a useful amount of new money available to fund the additional educational infrastructure needed in the medical schools for implementation.

David Shaw has now retired. I asked him recently why he thought the medical schools had responded positively to *Tomorrow's Doctors*. He was quite clear. There is no doubt that the inclusive discussions and the infrastructure money helped, but it was the knowledge that the GMC would check up on compliance, and that there could be consequences where that did not happen, that really mattered. That squares with my own experience. I asked the same question of a dean recently who said without hesitation 'because we knew that this time the GMC meant business'. Basic medical education in Britain today is regarded internationally as leading edge. It is one of the success stories of the NHS. All concerned can take pride in that. But the leadership for the changes that made that possible came from the Education Committee of the GMC at a time in the early nineties when regulation by the GMC seemed to be failing.

And the lessons were simple but vital in the story of the changing culture and the struggle to achieve it. Provide sound policy, present it attractively, explain it carefully and give scope for innovation and development, but provide sanctions, with a willingness to use them, should reason and persuasion fail.

Standards: good medical practice

In a three-year period of considerable activity (1993–95), the GMC was to revolutionise its ideas on professional culture and standards. The new thinking emerged from the Committee on Standards and Medical Ethics of the GMC that I chaired at that time. It was charged with giving ethical advice to the medical profession. Historically it did this through a little handbook of advice, the *'Blue Book'*,* which defined the kind of behaviours and conduct in a doctor which the GMC thought could constitute serious professional misconduct. It described how the GMC disciplined doctors. Thus it was the booklet used regularly by the PCC. Although it was given to every doctor on qualification, we suspected that most doctors did not read it because it was concerned with 'bad doctors.' If like the vast majority of doctors you considered yourself a 'good' doctor, it was not relevant to you.

Several factors in the late 1980s and early 1990s were stimulating change. For example, in 1984 we saw that, following the Alfie Winn case, guidance was given to the profession for the first time on good clinical care (*see* Chapter 6). Information to patients was becoming a public issue.

---

* The *Blue Book* – an abbreviation for *Professional Conduct and Discipline: fitness to practise.*

The Patients' Liaison Group of the RCGP was pressing for good information about the services of general practice available to patients. I was closely associated with that movement. Practice leaflets describing these services were soon to become a contractual requirement for NHS general practitioners. At about the same time the Monopolies and Mergers Commission taxed the GMC with opening up and removing restrictions on doctors' advertising. These two initiatives together caused considerable debate to which patients' organisations as well as doctors' contributed vigorously. There were divided reactions from the profession – some conservative, but others wanting to open up medicine. The consequence was that the Standards Committee recast its advice to doctors in a more positive form, emphasising the necessity for good information.

Another emerging standards issue was that of consent. Hitherto the GMC had taken the view that consent was a subject on which it was not qualified to give advice. It was essentially a legal matter. But views were changing, stimulated by several important cases before the PCC. The famous 'kidneys for sale' case in 1988 involved doctors Bewick, Crockett and Joyce with charges that included failure to establish that a patient understood adequately the risks, possible complications and after-effects of surgery.

A further stimulus came from *Tomorrow's Doctors*, just published. It focused on training. It did not set out to answer questions about the attributes of a doctor, and therefore what should be the outcome of university medical education. The idea of looking at the outcome of the educational process was quite novel, indeed revolutionary. The Standards Committee asked members of the Education Committee informally, 'What are the qualities of a good doctor?' The deans were no more able to answer that question than we were ourselves. We had a problem. If the GMC and the deans between them could not agree on the attributes of a good doctor, how could the profession know what was expected of it? How could there be reasonable consistency of outcome across the nation's medical schools? And how on earth would the public know whether the medical profession and the GMC had taken into account their expectations of a good doctor? Indeed, did we know what they wanted? This for me linked back to the RCGP's *Future General Practitioner*. The starting point of that whole process had been exactly the same – 'What is a good general practitioner?' We needed to know that in order to decide what had to be learned.

So, drawing these strands together, it became increasingly clear to my colleagues and I on the Standards Committee that the negatively framed *Blue Book* should be replaced by something more positive and inclusive. Could the *Blue Book* be revised, to make it more readable and its messages better retained?

By November 1994 any idea of a revision of the *Blue Book* had been abandoned as unrealistic and insufficient – it would be a case of new wine in old bottles. Instead we established a small Working Group* to look at questions afresh from first principles and with a clean sheet. From the start it was one of those small groups that was both exciting and creative. I felt we were really breaking new ground with new ideas with people who were really fired up to move the agenda on.

Patients had to be squarely at the centre of any new statement of professional values and standards. The message was to be about good doctoring, what it is and what duties and responsibilities a doctor has. The statement had to be simple, unambiguous and direct. It was to be inclusive, addressed to every registered doctor. In that spirit we decided to abandon the GMC's addiction to talking about the 'highest possible standards' – with all its élitist connotations – and to talk instead about 'good practice' which should be attainable by everybody on the medical register.

The Council felt that the statement should still be couched in terms of advice to the profession rather than as a set of requirements. Indeed there was quite a sharp debate about the distinction between 'should' and 'must.' Members were quick to point out that there seemed to be quite a few musts, for example in keeping up to date, in safe prescribing and so on. The idea of clinical audit as a required professional duty was rejected, which I thought was a mistake. (However, the decision was reversed in the 1998 revision of *Good Medical Practice*.) So in 1995 there were warning signs that, for some Council members at least, advice was fine so long as it was not binding. These reservations notwithstanding the Council was generally enthusiastic about the work and we were able to get agreement in May 1995 for publication.

The final product, *Good Medical Practice*,[52] was very simply written. The first part, on one page, stated the basic 'Duties of a Doctor', which are so important that I include them as Appendix A.† The second part – the booklet *Good Medical Practice* – described the principal attributes of good medical practice under the following main headings (taken from the revised 2001 version):

- Good clinical care
- Maintaining good medical practice

* The new group consisted of Professor Charles George, Dr John Havard (formerly Secretary of the BMA), Professor Ian Kennedy, Dr Michael O'Donnell, Professor Wendy Savage and myself in the chair. The group was supported by an outstanding staff member, Jane O'Brien.
† We were glad of Michael O'Donnell's help in drafting them. He had told me so often how much he disliked the *Blue Book* – a turn-off for anyone trying to read it. He had been keen since being elected to the GMC to have a go at rewriting it in English!

- Relationships with patients
- Teaching and training, appraising and assessing
- Working with colleagues
- Probity
- Health.

The initial reactions from both the profession and the public were favourable. *Good Medical Practice* told doctors clearly for the first time what was expected of them. And much feedback from non-doctors revealed a relief to see that the human aspects of medical care, which so many people felt the medical profession had forgotten about, were in fact all there.

I felt very positive about *Good Medical Practice*. With the important lay input there had been it was a consensus statement that brought professional and patient views on the qualities of a doctor together for the first time. It contained everything that was needed to change the culture of medicine in a direction properly in keeping with modern medical practice. It was the foundation of a new approach to professionalism in medicine.

The real challenge would be to make it stick wherever doctors carried GMC registration. Achieving compliance, as ever, would be the real test. As the Education Committee had discovered with its earlier guidance to medical schools, standards are virtually worthless unless people take notice of them. Later studies carried out by the GMC on the awareness of doctors of *Good Medical Practice* would confirm just how true this was.

Dealing with poor performance

In the early 1990s anxieties about poorly performing doctors continued to grow. Kenneth Calman brought representatives of the profession together, resulting in new guidance, *Maintaining Medical Excellence*,[53] in 1995. Liam Donaldson, then Regional Medical Officer in the Northern Region, analysed a substantial series of cases in his region.[54] The sociologist Marilynn Rosenthal had also been documenting patterns of poor performance in NHS practice in a series of studies.[55]

Meanwhile, after the long and laborious process that I described in Chapter 6, the President's Advisory Committee (PAC) decided to established a Working Group in May 1990 to develop procedures for dealing with serious deficiencies in a doctor's professional performance. The group, led by the President, Robert Kilpatrick, worked hard. After 17 meetings and a series of informal consultations with the profession and other interested parties, the group's report was presented to the Council, and accepted by the Council, in May 1992.

The performance procedures added a third arm to the existing committees dealing with professional conduct and health. They were modelled on the Health Committee procedures that were still relatively new and seemed to be working well. The purpose was primarily patient protection but there was equally the intention of restoring a poorly performing doctor to practice through remedial help wherever possible. The aim was to enable the Council to take action where complaints about a doctor's clinical performance over time suggested a pattern of serious deficiency. Where it was established that there appeared to be a pattern of poor performance the matter would be investigated and the evidence considered in a hearing, and then decisions made. Sanctions would include placing a restriction on a doctor's practice or suspending the doctor's registration. In procedural and process terms the thinking was quite conventional.

The discussions in the Working Group reflected the cultural climate of the time. In the GMC Council proceedings and in the medical press the tone was one of anxiety and protectiveness. There was high anxiety in the profession, particularly about any test of clinical knowledge or skill. General practitioners accepted the need for the proposed procedures more easily than specialists did. In the discussions with the BMA, I remember that Ian Bogle, who chaired the GMSC at that time, was in no doubt. But the specialists were less easily persuaded. At first their representatives felt that if there was a problem with a specialist's competence or performance it should be dealt with by the BMA or the relevant medical Royal College in consultation with the doctor's employer, using the employment contract arrangements. For them that system worked perfectly satisfactorily and so no GMC involvement was required. I was to remind Ian Bogle of this later, when we had to deal with that same BMA consultants' committee's hostile reactions to evidence-based revalidation.

It is a tribute to Robert Kilpatrick's persuasiveness with his specialist colleagues that they came round in due course to accept that poor performance could affect specialists as well as general practitioners, and that the new GMC procedures would have to apply to all doctors.

There then followed a further period of just over three years in attempting to get the proposals translated into legislation. Primary legislation was required and for that it was always difficult to find parliamentary time. Fortunately amongst the lay members the government had decided to appoint three MPs, one from each of the main political parties. Gareth Wardell (Labour) took up the cause with the Labour Opposition. Alex (now Lord) Carlisle brought in the Liberal Democrats, and both of them worked with the Conservative government to bring in the bill. Roger Sims (Conservative) was a lay screener on the GMC. He was able to speak persuasively in the Commons debate about his experience of dealing with complaints about poorly performing doctors. In December 1995 the Medical (Professional Performance) Act amended the 1993 Medical Act to include the new professional performance procedures.

The philosophy and the instruments

The really new thinking in the performance procedures was in the assessment process and the new assessment instruments. This was an important step forward. For the first time a doctor's overall performance would be assessed against explicit professional standards – indeed those being developed in *Good Medical Practice*. Performance was chosen becomes it comes closest to real practice. Doctors preferred that. 'Performance' describes what a doctor does in practice. 'Competence' describes the doctor's knowledge and skills. Clearly competence is subsumed within performance. A doctor can be knowledgeable but not apply that knowledge effectively in practice; but a doctor cannot perform well if not first competent.

Unlike the primarily paper-based tests of competence used in the United States and Canada, the GMC instruments were designed to assess the performance of the doctor at work. Formal written tests of competence were to follow in a second phase where a problem was identified.

The decision to use performance as the definitive measure was based on the extensive experience gained in general practice through the RCGP membership examination and *Fellowship by Assessment*. So it was not surprising that Robert Kilpatrick invited Professor (now Dame) Lesley Southgate, the Chief Examiner of the RCGP, to lead the group on method development. It was Lesley's job to assemble an expert technical team, drawn from all specialities, to establish a set of core methods and instruments that would give a comprehensive and reliable insight into a doctor's practice. The work began in 1994 and was essentially completed when the procedures became operational in 1997. She and her colleagues, drawn mainly from the medical Royal Colleges, produced an outstanding piece of work, details of which, in terms of methods and studies of their implementation, were published later.[56]

The design required that assessments of performance at the workplace would be carried out by a team of two medical assessors from the same discipline as the doctor (one of whom would be in clinical practice similar to that of the doctor) and a lay assessor. A medical assessor would lead the team. All assessors were to be trained. The GMC made a point from the outset that lay and medical members would learn together – a good example of practical multidisciplinary learning. At the workplace the assessors were to systematically collect and document evidence against a sampling framework derived from an assessment blueprint. Although they would conduct some assessments together, each assessor would see a different sample at the doctor's practice because they would follow different programmes during the visit. There would be many samples of the doctor's practice available and many cross-checks. If the assessors were not satisfied, the doctor's knowledge and clinical skills might be tested, using a variety of instruments designed for the purpose.

These methods represented a major step forward in handling poor performance and have attracted serious international interest. Used within a legal framework and accepted by the profession and the public alike, they ultimately provided the foundation for revalidation.

Losing the plot: what was not done

Now we come to the downside of the curate's egg. Despite the new developments, the Council like the profession it reflected was still struggling to come to terms with medical practice in a society that was changing. The workings of the Council itself exemplified this, as I describe later. Even at this stage it was still completely wedded to its traditional piecemeal approach to medical regulation that was becoming more anachronistic by the day. It still worked in a world of its own. There was still a strong clubby atmosphere. The building itself at 44 Hallam Street looked like a London club. There was dark wood panelling, leather chairs, a staff deferential to members and good lunches. There was a standing joke that the GMC ran round lunch. A meeting would be arranged in the afternoon, beginning with lunch or would be held in the morning, to conclude with lunch. The first week I became President, I was told that at the start of each week I had to agree the lunch menus for everyone who would come to the GMC that week. Changing that was one of my first decisions!

The GMC of that time did not see itself, nor did others see it, as a mainstream player in medical care. It did not look at the big picture of developing quality and the nature of medical practice, and ask itself what as the regulator it could and should contribute to that. It did not scan the horizon, think in terms of health policy development or check its own functions against changes going on around it. It did not automatically think 'patients'. In business terms it did not really know what business it was in, and so had no real idea of where it should go. Indeed, two former senior civil servants have told me that the BMA and the medical Royal Colleges scarcely mentioned it in their discussions with government. And the DoH for its part saw it simply as the body that dealt with doctors' ethical misconduct. Robert Kilpatrick tried to rectify this by setting up a strategic review in 1991. This failed because most time was spent on descriptive reviews of committee business. A mission statement did emerge but it was meaningless without the will, capacity and understanding of the need for strategic thinking. Modern, customer-friendly, quality-driven management methods were not in the mindset, not in the culture of the Council nor in the staff organisation supporting it.

The large size of the Council lent itself to this piecemeal approach. So the Council divided its work into little boxes. Thus for example education was, metaphorically speaking, walled off on its own, the province of the medical school deans tempered by input from a few non-academic doctors and lay members. There were separate arrangements for overseas doctors in their own box with its own outlook and its own systems. The Registration Committee, responsible for the integrity of the Medical Register, functioned essentially as a bureaucratic process, not central to the maintenance of quality in the profession. The Fitness to Practise Committees, of which the Professional Conduct Committee was the most public face of the GMC, functioned through a series of panels on which members were elected to serve. But most members had little idea of how the disciplinary function related to the wider issues of professionalism – how could they? The Executive Committee, later rebadged as the President's Advisory Committee, had no clearly defined policy development role, so it tended to deal with the day-to-day affairs that did not fit into a functioning committee brief.

There was a clear separation between 'the Council' concerned with policy, and the permanent staff of the organisation charged with the delivery of the services to implement that policy. Members were expected to deal with policy matters that were presented to them. The functioning of the organisation was not seen as their responsibility. This could create tension with committee chairs when they complained, for example, about the staff's style of letter writing on their behalf or the slowness in getting correspondence answered.

Consequently members, and therefore everybody else, knew very little about the staff organisation that lay behind the GMC. It was led by a Registrar who was by custom recruited from the Civil Service. The President and the Registrar together were really responsible for its shape and character. Thus Robert Kilpatrick had a close working relationship with Peter Towers, the Registrar. When a new Registrar was appointed in 1994 – Finlay Scott, another Civil Servant – the opportunity was taken to restyle the post 'Chief Executive' and Registrar, and to make him more clearly responsible for the functioning of the organisation – 'the office' as he called it. I thought that a Chief Executive who would modernise the management of the GMC's services would be absolutely vital.

The new Registrar was appointed to start making the much needed changes. The processes were very old-fashioned, like the Civil Service in the early 1950s – shades of Sir Humphrey!* Little things illustrate the culture of the 1980s and early 1990s. For example, I remember wanting to fax a document to the GMC from my own home. That was a problem because the GMC did not have a machine at that time. I was told I could fax my papers to the GMC's lawyers, who were in a separate building, and the GMC would 'send a runner' to collect them! Another example was the extremely difficult telephone access via the GMC switchboard. Council members complained they could not get through to the GMC on the telephone, so to resolve this a new direct line for members was installed. Of course this ignored the fact that the rest of the world – the customers – still had an access problem! And so it went on.

It is easy to mock these limitations. But one has to see the GMC then as an organisation in a time warp. Members came together twice a year for Council meetings. They were by and large busy people with their main jobs in life elsewhere. Many of the medical members of this large governing body had their principal professional allegiances outside the Council – to their College, the BMA or other organisations, not to the GMC. So beyond the President, the Registrar and to a limited degree the committee chairs, members had no real motivation or incentive to take appropriate collective responsibility for the functioning of the organisation in its day-to-day business of investigating complaints, conducting hearings, checking credentials of doctors seeking registration and so on. Indeed they were not encouraged to – members were members and staff were staff.

As well as its introspection, remoteness and lack of responsiveness, the GMC already had a reputation at that stage for being hopelessly slow with its Fitness to Practise administrative procedures, particularly in the Fitness to Practise Division. There was an established 'backlog' culture that was to become the millstone that would nearly sink the organisation. Complainants were frustrated by the GMC's slowness and perceived unwillingness to deal with any but the most severe of cases. Doctors from overseas seeking registration found the processes very bureaucratic and slow. NHS managers, increasingly aware of their vulnerability when confronted with dysfunctional doctors, were equally critical. These criticisms seldom surfaced in any concrete or organised way, and ominously they did not filter through to the members because there was no properly constituted mechanism for dealing with 'customer' complaints. Indeed the GMC did not understand the concept of 'customer' at all, despite the consumer revolution going on around it.

Another deep-seated cultural characteristic was the lack of transparency in its processes. This manifested itself in all sorts of ways. The

---

* Sir Humphrey Appleby, the fictional Permanent Secretary and then Cabinet Secretary in the BBC series *Yes, Minister* and *Yes, Prime Minister*, played by Nigel Hawthorne.

organisation, like many others at the time, was itself very secretive – 'never give any information not absolutely necessary.' But this secrecy affected member processes as well. The screening of complaints, for example, was a process that was completely hidden. Then again for many years the PCC did not think it appropriate to give any explanation for its decisions. Yet another bizarre example, which I discovered only recently, was the office practice in the 1970s of secretaries preventing members of the public from getting copies of the *Blue Book*, the advice on misconduct, in the belief that it might stimulate ideas for complaints about doctors.

So the GMC was a slow, rule-dominated, reactive organisation in which no one was truly accountable for its operational processes. It positively resisted transparency. It had a hand-to-mouth existence. It was driven by complaints and it gave the strong impression, through the way in which it conducted its business, of not wishing to be involved in wider matters except as a last resort.

It would be wrong to give the impression that individual members and members of staff were unconcerned about the situation. Indeed the new Registrar and his team and a growing number of members were. But it was difficult to find a way in, to get to grips with the problem. It was like wrestling with a jellyfish – you thought you had hold of it, then it would slip away. The forces for maintaining the *status quo*, both members and staff, were very strong.

The sense of inertia was reinforced by the professional organisations. As we have seen the universities took little notice of what the Education Committee did, until the latter showed its mettle with *Tomorrow's Doctors*. The medical Royal Colleges were most interested in making sure that the GMC did not stray seriously into their territory, into specialist training or CPD, or indeed even act decisively on its statutory duty to co-ordinate all stages of medical education. The BMA, which wanted no interference from the GMC with its direct interest in professional regulation through NHS contracts, was not pressing hard on the criticisms raised by Richard Smith in the *BMJ*, all of which reflected what I have described. All in all the medical stakeholders still gave the impression that they wanted a GMC which would not make waves, and not intrude on their territory except in those circumstances where a doctor was behaving in a way that by general consent 'let the side down.' The *status quo* again.

Ordinary doctors did not want the GMC intruding on their lives. Most were as ignorant about its full range of functions as were ordinary members of the public. For this, the GMC had only itself to blame. But then it did not mind because its perceptions of its role were minimalist anyway.

All this was consistent with the picture revealed at the 'summit' meeting of the profession in 1994 to which I referred in Chapter 1. That meeting, to consider the core values of the profession and whether they needed changing, had been prompted by the CMO, Kenneth Calman. At about that time, he had set out his ideas on modern professionalism, with which I very much agreed.[3] At the meeting there were some excellent papers and it was a good initiative. But behind the papers the discussions that I attended revealed strongly defensive attitudes and very little insight into the profound nature of the social changes that had already happened all around us. I was struck forcibly by the fact that patients were not seriously involved in that conference. It was a profession – and a BMA – still looking inwardly at itself. Despite all the warnings, it was not getting the message about the need to strengthen self-regulation.

Meanwhile, Richard Smith[57] continued to question the willingness and capacity of the GMC to put self-regulation on a sound basis. He used leaders in the *BMJ* to try to raise awareness and energy levels, to increase the sense of urgency. In 1993 he said:

> Time may be running out for the GMC. Well into its second century, it is trying to come up with a recipe for dealing with doctors who perform consistently poorly. The [GMC's] ideas have been several years in the making and are at least three to four years from implementation. The risk to the Council is that it fails to produce a system that satisfies both doctors and the public or that its painfully slow procedures are overtaken by speedier events – like a scandalous case or a political campaign to substitute self-regulation with regulation by the State.

These words were written just three years before the situation at Bristol – a 'scandalous case' – broke.

He added later that year in another editorial:[58]

> Not with a bang but with a whimper, the GMC is slipping into history . . . The government is sidelining the GMC and with it the self-regulation the profession has enjoyed since 1858.

Part 3
Making progress, making waves

8

Leading from the front

In May 1995 there was a Council election for a new President. Robert Kilpatrick was stepping down after some six years in office. My interest in the job was motivated primarily by what I thought the GMC now needed to do to play its part in developing and implementing modern ideas on professionalism and professional regulation. I decided to stand for election therefore on a manifesto for radical reform. I believed that the GMC should be leading change in the profession and in itself energetically and positively. I was an enthusiastic supporter of the new developments in medical education, the performance procedures and professional standards described in Chapter 7. Nevertheless I shared the view of Margaret Stacey, Richard Smith and others that these developments of themselves were insufficient, and the pace of change too slow, to take the public and the medical profession into a new, stable relationship of respect and trust.

In the election there were four candidates. Sir Herbert Duthie was an appointed member from the University of Wales and a much respected Chairman of the PCC. Sir Anthony Grabham had been the Chairman of Council of the BMA and was now a senior BMA figure. Beulah Bewley, the only female candidate, was a Treasurer of the GMC, formerly very active in the Medical Women's Federation, and very keen on the purchase of a modern building. And myself.

For the first time candidates were asked to offer an election statement on two sides of A4 paper. My supporters and I decided on a bold, forward-looking election address, based on a strongly patient-oriented philosophy. My primary objective was the implementation of the professional standards set out in *Good Medical Practice* across the practising profession. It needed to be done in a way that would 'touch the hearts and engage the minds . . . so that doctors and medical students feel a sense of ownership and commitment which is reflected in their everyday work'.

As to the GMC, I wanted it to lead from the front on internal reform based on the principles of quality improvement and quality assurance. I sought a GMC that would be proactive rather than only reactive to complaints. I wanted it to listen to and be responsive to all its stake-holders, not just the doctors, to think strategically and to publish its work regularly in ways that would give everyone a clear account of its activities and its effectiveness. As a test of its resolve I was determined that the pre-registration year – still essentially unchanged despite the Merrison recommendation for improvement 20 years earlier – would at last be modernised to give every new doctor a well-taught, properly supervised and enjoyable start to a career in medicine. Overall my aim was a GMC founded on modern principles of regulation, 'a model of excellence amongst regulating bodies' based on 'good standards and demonstrably reliable performance'.

Some said that this upfront approach was risky in an election. It may have been, but so far as I was concerned if the mood were to proceed slowly or to preserve the *status quo*, I would be the wrong person. I was not interested in the job for the sake of it.

In the event the election results revealed a clear though not over-whelming win. I was the first general practitioner in the 137 years of the GMC's history to hold the office of President. I knew that my support came from all sections of the Council electorate and that it was particularly strong with lay members, so there was no tribalism in it. The election reckoning suggested that just over half the members wanted serious change, and so I felt justified in interpreting the result as a mandate for reform.

Some elected members felt strongly that the President should come from the elected member constituency, because all previous Presidents had been drawn from the members appointed by the universities and medical Royal Colleges, as I was. I knew, therefore, how disappointed the BMA would be that Sir Anthony had not been chosen. Sandy Macara, the then Chairman of the BMA Council, told me just prior to the election in a meal together that I ought to stand aside, to give Sir Anthony a clear run. He said that I would be defeated if I persisted. That served only to make me even more determined, and not to be intimidated. I never believed that Sir Anthony had been party to this pressure and indeed I had cast-iron support subsequently from both him and my other two colleagues who had stood for election. They all buckled into the reform programme with a will, whatever reservations they themselves may have had privately.

Getting started

My presidency began on 1 September 1995. The Council was in good heart. It had not yet become aware of the unfolding situation at the Bristol

Royal Infirmary, although clearly some members with local connections must have known of it. The Medical (Professional Performance) Bill had just been enacted, paving the way for the introduction of our performance procedures. *Good Medical Practice* had just been published and had been well received by both the profession and patients' organisations. And the reports from the universities about progress in implementing *Tomorrow's Doctors* were extremely satisfying and encouraging. The main clouds on the horizon for Council members were real anxieties about the charge of racism within the GMC in connection with the investigation of complaints against overseas-qualified doctors. The GMC was looking into this through a group chaired by Rani Atma, a lay member.

Nevertheless, dangers were piling up ahead for the profession and the GMC. My sense of urgency about the need for speedy reform received a strong shot in the arm in those first three months between September 1995 and the end of the year. I met representatives of consumer and patient interests* because I wanted to hear at firsthand what they thought. I wanted to make the point, at the very outset, that the GMC under my leadership was going to deal with the public as a full stakeholder.

In our conversations they painted a picture of the GMC – a reflection of the medical profession as seen through consumer eyes – that was far from reassuring. They knew all about the awkward attitudes of some doctors, especially about the handling of complaints, and what they considered to be a lack of a sense of proper accountability within the profession. There were serious criticisms about the performance of the GMC as an organisation, especially in the screening of patients' complaints, which was regarded as being deadly slow, loaded against the complainant, bureaucratic and seriously lacking in transparency. Arnold Simanovitz, for example, was critical of the GMC for its stubbornly reactive stance to problems of poor practice. He believed that if it became aware of a problem it should itself (or cause others) to initiate investigations without waiting for a formal complaint. Similarly patients, unlike doctors, had no right of appeal against GMC decisions arising from complaints. And too often decisions, especially in cases involving clinical care, appeared to favour the doctor rather than the patients. Set against these serious criticisms, what the GMC saw as major strides forward in education, performance and standard setting, whilst welcome, seemed less impressive to them.

---

* Those people included Linda Lamont from the Patients' Association, Marion Rigge from the College of Health, Brian Yates and Derek Prentice from the Consumers' Association, Toby Harris representing Community Health Councils, Helena Shovelton from the Citizens Advice Bureau and Arnold Simanovitz from the Association for the Victims of Medical Accidents. Most I had met previously, and knew some well. I had kept in touch with Ian Kennedy, and I knew how people like Robert Maxwell (then Chief Executive of the King's Fund), Rudolph Klein and Barbara Stocking (then also at the King's Fund) all felt.

This preliminary reconnaissance, the assessment of the state of the organisation made by Finlay Scott, the new Chief Executive, and my own observations on the functioning of the GMC reinforced in my mind that, despite the good progress on the three big policy developments, the GMC was still nevertheless not in a fit shape to protect the public properly or to safeguard the good name of the profession. We both recognised that there was a huge mountain to climb.

The strategy

It was important that we were all clear about a common direction and purpose. I had led change on other occasions and had learnt how vital this was. I set out my approach in two major public lectures, the Haliburton-Hume in Newcastle upon Tyne in March 1996 and the Telford Lecture at the Manchester Medical Society later that year. These were distilled in two papers published by the *BMJ* in May 1997.[6,7] (I have always found the discipline of writing essential to the development and clear presentation of ideas.) They and later lectures had three purposes – indicating the direction of travel I thought we should follow, the development of ideas on strategic policy and providing the opportunity for subjecting these ideas to wide exposure and scrutiny.

The nub was simply this. Patients and doctors have a common interest in effective medical professionalism backed by effective professionally led regulation. Doctors' personal professionalism must be based in future on their observance of explicit professional standards agreed between the profession and the public (the new *Good Medical Practice*). There must be robust arrangements to secure full and willing compliance throughout a doctor's active professional life. The standards must be embedded in medical education so that doctors in training absorb the culture from their earliest days.

The culture of standard setting, quality improvement and quality assurance should extend equally to clinical teams throughout the NHS and private sector, and in institutions like the GMC. It should become a fundamental part of everyday professional life. I explained how this might be done through evidence-based medicine, regular audit, regular appraisal and so on.

I believed that the medical culture was predicated on a number of propositions. All doctors and clinical teams had a duty to maintain and demonstrate good practice. Collectively, public involvement in professional regulation was essential. Professional self-regulation is a privilege, not a right. Therefore effective accountability must be built into the system at all levels – GMC, hospitals and general practice, clinical teams and for individual doctors. Openness about doctors' performance both at the local and institutional levels was essential for public trust.

Patients must be protected from poor practice. Poorly performing doctors should be helped back to practice wherever possible.

I said that in the UK we had got professional regulation the wrong way round. The emphasis was all on centrally driven, complaints-activated machinery built around the GMC. But if dysfunctional practice was to be prevented or, when it occurred, to be detected and acted upon early, the emphasis in future must be on local systems and particularly local quality assurance in clinical teams with any central machinery there as a back-up.

So the key elements of a new model of professional regulation were clear in my mind. These ideas were developed subsequently in a series of papers in the *Lancet*,[15,59] and, following the Lloyds Robert lecture in January 2000, in the *Journal of the Royal Society of Medicine* (RSM).[60] The advantage of personal papers was that they promoted feedback and reaction without committing the organisation prematurely. They were my contribution to the pool of ideas swirling around about the way forward for the medical profession.

Implementation

To implement reform there needed to be action on two fronts. One was external with the profession, patients' organisations, government, universities and so on. The other was internal, particularly with the processes and internal structure of the GMC that clearly needed attention. Finlay Scott and I agreed a basic division of effort. As Chief Executive he would be responsible for sorting out the functioning of the GMC internal organisation. As President, although I had overall responsibility for strategy and implementation, I would concentrate on leading change with the profession.

In Chapter 2 I described the methods used in the Northern Region training practices to introduce consensus professional standards and to embed them in the training practice culture. It required hard, dedicated work by a lot of people. It had to be sustained and so it required infrastructure. Above all it required leadership. There is all the difference in the world between a 'tick box' approach with minimum investment in commitment, and securing and maintaining the wholehearted engagement of people who are doing something they believe in. It's rather like the difference between a check-list approach to gaining patients' consent to treatment – quick and easy – compared with the effort needed over time to achieve the understanding necessary for true, fully informed consent. The task now was to get the over 100 000 doctors working in the UK to sign up, just like the trainers. The task was the same but with a completely different order of magnitude.

Nevertheless I felt that the same basic principles should apply in getting the principles of *Good Medical Practice* accepted and practised by doctors. Breaking the profession down into identifiable, manageable groups that would take ownership would be a basic step. Leaders would be crucial. Hence the decision to look from the outset to more robust alliances. The medical schools had already demonstrated leadership in the implementation of *Tomorrow's Doctors*. Equally important were the certificating bodies for training (the STA and JCPTGP). The medical Royal Colleges themselves broke down into much smaller, cohesive subspeciality groupings through specialist societies and they shared with the GMC the main responsibility for professional standards. Similarly early on I asked the BMA, through its then Chairman Sandy Macara, to see if their local structures could help strengthen local medical regulation. And there were early discussions with the NHS about raising employer awareness of the qualities expected of a doctor in *Good Medical Practice*, for example when making consultant appointments and in decisions about distinction awards.

This dispersed approach through many different groups meant that to manage change with any hope of success, in addition to the alliances, I would have to be a travelling President. I needed to be able to listen to people, to discuss and argue with them directly. This is how I had learnt to lead the general practitioner trainers and RCGP members both when I was Honorary Secretary and later as Chairman of Council. I used the medium of lectures, talks and seminars to test the thinking on policy and to share that with all the relevant stakeholders. In the course of six years I met several thousand people – doctors, patients, the well public, managers and other health professionals.

To pursue the partnership idea, I visited every medical school and medical Royal College to talk about what they could do to get the values of *Good Medical Practice* embedded into the learning culture and into assessments. As I had learnt in general practice, getting the teachers signed up was a vital first step – they became the leaders. And so during the medical school visits – usually two-day affairs – we talked about clinical teachers as role models of good practice, giving leadership by example within their own specialities and clinical teams. I specifically asked to meet representatives of patients' organisations, and the chairs, chief executives and non-executive trust board members, as well as medical teachers and students. I wanted to hear their views about medical training and the regulation of doctors, and what they could do to help. On more than one occasion I found myself acting, inadvertently, as a kind of neutral facilitator when round-table conversations touched on sensitive areas that clearly everybody knew about but had not apparently felt able to talk about openly before. Examples included big subjects like how education and service managers, each with responsibilities that were central for them, could help each other rather than compete. And there were particular issues, for example, about how new doctors would learn to explain to patients about errors and handle difficult colleagues. The difficult questions were invariably about attitudes and relationships. At times doctors, patients and managers had quite different views.

I tried to make sure that the consumer/patients' viewpoint was always heard. I had learnt that the presence of lay public members always altered the dynamics of conversation, whether in a group or over dinner. It stopped doctors – and managers – talking only to themselves. Of course there was another purpose to this too. It was to expose to them the view of the GMC as a regulator which was interested in, and contributed positively to, the quality of healthcare as well as the educational and disciplinary functions with which they were all familiar.

Fortunately I was able to travel and speak in the confidence that my colleagues would be sharing the load, and contributing hugely to policy development. I provided the sense of direction – the vision if you like – but nothing would have been achieved without a strong team to challenge, refine, amend, develop, restrain where necessary and implement. For example, members and staff* together ran highly successful road shows around the regions about the new performance procedures. Doctors, the public and NHS managers were the audience. What we learnt was how much we needed to hear about how it was for people on the ground, and what we needed to do to make the new processes for handling poorly performing doctors useful to them.

Meanwhile throughout my term we continued to build relationships with the patient and consumer interests. We secured the help of the King's Fund and Nuffield Trust as independent agencies with no axe to grind, on some practical aspects of policy development. And latterly arising from the discussions on revalidation, we established a standing GMC Patients' Reference Group that was led by a very committed and able lay member, Sue Leggate.

Within the GMC we used the medium of small-group discussion – members' seminars – to work through ideas on the big subjects, for example governance, fitness to practise, reform and revalidation. These were a critical part of the process. The Council as a single body was far too big for that kind of effective working up and exchange of views. The GMC itself published in due course major policy papers on revalidation, the constitution and governance of the GMC, and on the redesign of the Fitness to Practise procedures. This proactive approach enabled us in the GMC to disseminate ideas about the unfolding agenda through what one

---

* Alan Howes was the staff member who led the performance work with great dedication.

might call 'think-pieces', papers exploring ideas in advance of policy papers for formal consultation.

So that was broadly how we approached the task, but things rarely go quite as planned.

Events dear boy, events*

In driving change I expected increasing pressure from outside. I believed that when the new performance procedures kicked in, a considerable reservoir of poor or inadequate general practice – that as we have seen many people knew about – would be exposed to the light of day. That would raise questions. I did not expect anything like the same effect from hospital practice. Which just goes to show how wrong you can be. 'Events dear boy, events', as Harold Macmillan ruefully put it.

The events at Bristol Royal Infirmary first surfaced in my radar in April 1996 when William Rees Mogg wrote about it in *The Times*. Bristol and its aftermath was to dominate the whole of my presidency. Bristol, and the other small collection of very high-profile cases which all came to public notice at about the same time, became the key drivers of change. We, the public, decided that up with more of this we would not put. What started as a loss of confidence in doctors and particularly their regulator, the GMC, soon spread to become part of a much wider national debate about the overall performance of the NHS, and indeed public services generally.

In the six years between 1996 and the end of 2001 a new model of standards-driven professional regulation was developed and agreed. The GMC retained responsibility for leading and managing the change process, even though at one point it looked as if it would founder under the huge external and often conflicting pressures that came to bear. By the end of 2002 Parliament had agreed the new framework to which all stakeholders – public, profession and employers – had signed up.

The remainder of this book is about how that change came about. There were two distinct phases. The first, from 1996 to June 1998 when the case against the Bristol doctors ended, was relatively calm. Then the pace of change accelerated tremendously until, after a battle between the GMC and some parts of the profession, there was resolution in November 2001.

---

* Attributed to Harold Macmillan when asked what his biggest problem was.

In the rest of this chapter I want to set the scene by mentioning the various drivers for change. In a way they provided the context, and then I shall illustrate some of the cultural changes within the GMC itself.

Drivers for change

There were five main players – the public, the government, the profession, the press and the law.

The public

I have described the public reaction to the high-profile cases as the main driver. Public reaction made itself felt through the media (or sometimes it felt that the media provoked and stoked public reaction!), through Members of Parliament and in creating a climate in everyday life. Basically the public view was that enough was enough, and something had to be done.

There were local foci of pressure associated with the individual cases. In most of the big cases, patient action groups emerged. These became a new and powerful force: the Bristol parents, the parents of the children at Alder Hey, the patients of Rodney Ledward and Richard Neale, the bereaved families of patients murdered by Harold Shipman, and many others less publicly known, all helped by their actions to concentrate minds on their need for action to prevent future damage to others and when errors occur for proper explanations and apologies where appropriate. These action groups soon established communications with each other and with others overseas. They were very effective. They represented a new force that in my opinion has been helpful overall.

Slightly different were the consumer groups. The National Consumer Council (NCC), the Consumers' Association (CA) and the Patients' Association were perhaps the most powerful because of their thoughtful and practical contributions to improving professional regulation. The many organisations there are for patients with specific diseases added their distinctive perspectives by letting doctors see how patients with particular conditions felt, and what they expected. Smaller and highly focused was the Action for Victims of Medical Accidents (AVMA), the College of Health and Patient Concern. And in a more general way, the Community Health Councils and Citizens Advice Bureaux that had tremendous practical experience of the things that patients worried or complained about added their weight.

The government

I include the NHS because they seem inseparable. Government policy, both Conservative and Labour, was to be a huge driver, partly because government thought change right anyway, and partly in response to public pressure. I return to this below.

The profession

It may be that the stance of the medical profession appeared wholly reactive but this was not so. The role of the profession as a driver of change itself is part of the story.

The press

The press had a huge influence, for good or ill, depending on one's point of view. The press certainly provided focus in reporting on doctors appearing before the GMC. Specific investigations highlighted areas where public expectation and current practice were apart, for example on the GMC's policies on the restoration to the register of doctors who had been struck off. Editorial comment added weight in helping to shape and present the public view. Much of the case reporting I found accurate. But doctors often felt strongly about the one-sidedness and perceived unfairness when the charges against a doctor attracted lurid headlines, but the defence, especially when there was an acquittal, did not. In the big cases in particular – Bristol is a good example – the question of trial by the media became a real issue.

The law

The judiciary were a very specialised, discrete force for change through their attitudes to medical litigation. Essentially the courts became less deferential to doctors. Hence, for example, the assertive questioning of what was meant by reasonable practice in medical negligence cases and, in the case of the Fitness to Practise committees of the GMC – and all other regulators of health professionals – a much greater tendency to question the decisions of panels hearing cases which were appealed. Isabel Nisbet, Director of Policy at the GMC, recently completed an excellent study of doctors' appeals to the Privy Council, highlighting the changing attitudes reflected in their adjudication.

They contributed to the cultural change in process also. All the health regulators have been required to improve the transparency of the proceedings by, for example, giving appropriate explanations of their determinations. Lastly the new Human Rights Act legislation came into force in 2000, setting new standards of fairness of process. It required all existing legislation – including all the GMC's rules and regulations – to be interpreted in the light of the Act.

A new political era

Governments are powerful drivers of change. I want next to summarise government action in the second half of the 1990s because it provides essential context. In the previous chapter we saw the effect of the early Conservative administrations in changing heathcare. However, in the mid-1990s the mood of the country was changing and a strong tide was beginning to run in favour of a change of government. The Conservative government under John Major had rowed back somewhat from the sharper edges of the internal market. But despite this, the lack of goodwill and feeling for government policy on health was widespread both within the professions, within health service management and of course in the opposition political parties. It was against that background that the then Secretary of State, Stephen Dorrell, produced what were to be the Conservative government's final papers on health.

The White Paper on Primary Care was very developmental. The more general policy paper, *A Service with Ambitions* (November 1996),[61] was I thought one of the best policy papers that the Conservatives produced. It was the brainchild of Stephen Dorrell, ably helped by Alan Langlands, the Chief Executive of the NHS, Ken Calman, the CMO and Yvonne Moores, the Chief Nursing Officer (CNO). It was deeply patient-oriented – there could be no mistake that the days of the producer-dominated culture in the NHS were over – and positively developmental in its approach.

But in the event these last minute efforts were to no avail. A Labour government was elected with an overwhelming majority in May 1997. The style of the new administration was completely different. I met Frank Dobson and most of his ministerial team within the first week of their taking office. We were soon to learn that, as an insider said, 'this lot are completely different'. The New Labour administration was much more independent-minded about where it got its advice and ideas. So, we were to discover that it would not consult with the profession in the usual way. Senior civil servants felt marginalised. The new government used its completely independent lines of advice through its own policy advisors, built up whilst in opposition, and its network of focus groups. This is all very obvious now but it was actually quite a shock when we all started to adjust to the new reality in 1997.

Meanwhile, both the outgoing Conservative and incoming Labour governments were getting to grips with the growing crisis around the safety and quality of clinical care. The chronology is important. At Bristol the crisis in paediatric cardiac surgery had been reached in January 1995 with the death of a child, Joshua Loveday. In February 1995 Rodney Ledward was suspended by his NHS trust, and would be gone – dismissed – by December. Soon police investigations would begin into Harold Shipman, leading to his arrest in September 1998. Although none of this was hitting the headlines fully yet, the new government was fully briefed by the end of its first month in office on all serious clinical cases known to be emerging. The systems defects revealed through these cases both in regulation and the functioning of the NHS had an important bearing on the shape of the new legislation to come.

New Labour continued with the strong patient orientation – there was all-party consensus on that – but in due course it raised the whole game on quality, the development of which was welcome news to me. I said so to Frank Dobson when I told him about our determination in the GMC to modernise professional self-regulation for medicine.

Bristol and Ledward, when taken in conjunction with problems in several other centres, inevitably brought media focus on the medical profession in general and the GMC in particular. Despite the reassuring words in the House of Commons with the passage of the Medical (Professional Performance) Bill, there were nevertheless dissenting voices in Parliament that had no confidence in professional self-regulation or the GMC.

Clinical quality

In December 1997 the government introduced its new White Paper *The New NHS: modern, dependable*.[62] This reflected its determination that patients should be at the heart of its reforms, so reinforcing the foundations laid by the Thatcher and Major administrations. The internal market as such was to be abolished but the purchaser/provider split and NHS trusts were retained. Quality was to be the driving ethos.

A further White Paper, *A First-class Service*,[63] came out in June 1998. This was an excellent document that put quality fairly and squarely on the future agenda for the NHS in England, though the principles were expected to apply across the UK. 'The new NHS will have quality at its heart' seemed to signal the message and the priority to be given to it. The approach was the classic standards model – setting clear national service standards, disseminating these and monitoring compliance – familiar stuff.

In England, the National Institute for Clinical Excellence (NICE) was established with the job of developing evidence-based clinical guidelines on all aspects of healthcare and its delivery, and assessing and evaluating new technologies that might be used in the NHS. Complementing these national clinical guidelines, National Service Frameworks (NSF) were created to map out the essential ingredients of good clinical service provision. Originally there were three – for coronary heart disease, cancer and mental health. Following the Bristol case another was added for paediatric care.

Delivery was to be grounded on what Liam Donaldson christened 'clinical governance'. This was defined as 'a framework through which NHS organisations are accountable for continuously improving the quality of their services and safeguarding standardised care by creating an environment in which excellence in clinical care can flourish'. I saw it essentially as the application of good management practice to the clinical process. Underpinning clinical governance there would be lifelong learning and modern self-regulation.

To monitor implementation, the government established in England the Commission for Health Improvement (CHI), charged with carrying out inspections of all institutions across the NHS to check on the sufficiency of clinical governance and of compliance with the NICE standards. In 2002, after two years of operation, the government extended its remit to include private hospitals in external audit. So it became the independent Commission for Health Audit and Inspection (CHAI). The National Patient Safety Agency (NPSA) was established to monitor issues to do with patient safety.[64] In keeping with modern thinking on risk management, the system has been modelled along the aviation industry's machinery for reporting 'near misses'. And more recently, in January 2003, the Commission for Patient and Public Involvement in Health was established, together with Patients' Forums, to champion and promote the involvement of the public in local health services.

There was a particular emphasis on the poorly performing doctor. As a result of a consultation paper prepared by the CMO,[65] the National Clinical Assessment Authority (NCAA) was established in England to support NHS management. This was controversial at first, until its mode of working was fully worked out. It provides for the local assessment and retraining of poorly performing doctors, complementing the GMC centrally which deals with severe cases when a doctor's registration may be in question.

And lastly, following the recommendation of the Kennedy Report[1] on Bristol, a new overarching body for the individual health professions – the Council for the Regulation of Health Professionals (CRHP) – was established to co-ordinate and harmonise the work of the regulators of each of the health professions. It was given reserve powers, to be used only with parliamentary consent, to order individual regulators to change their rules.

Similar arrangements were made in Scotland although, with devolution, the Scots had clear ideas of their own as to how to achieve the common objective. For example, the Clinical Standards Board in Scotland brought together within one body the functions undertaken by NICE and the CHI in England. It built on the work of the Royal Colleges in Scotland, which were far better co-ordinated in creating clinical guidelines – the SIGN guidelines – than their counterparts in England.

The NHS Plan[66] was announced in 2000. It included a Modernisation Agency to take forward the detailed work, particularly the implementation of clinical governance. Part of the plan included new contractual obligations for all NHS doctors, for the first time, to have their clinical work appraised annually by their peers.

In terms of regulation the government's thinking concentrated initially on the NHS – it had an ideological dislike of the private sector and shut it out of sight. But as capacity problems in the NHS became more pressing, and some instances of poor practice in the private sector came to light, the thinking moved on to extend the regulatory framework to the private sector, and indeed to foster public–private partnerships in the provision of healthcare.

Two other points are important. First, in 1997 Frank Dobson placed a duty of quality on the chief executives of NHS trusts. This meant that it would be clear in future where the responsibility for service quality in a hospital would lie.

Second, part of *The NHS Plan* was the reform of the regulators of the health professions – all of them. The government produced proposals for the nursing profession and the professions allied to medicine in what it considered to be a blueprint for all professions. The medical profession's emerging new thinking about the culture of professionalism and its regulation was not evident to anything like the same extent in the other health professions. Nor was there much evidence of new policy thinking, particularly on the critical issues around professionalism, in the government's own proposals for individual health profession regulation, beyond structures, public representation, accountability and some curiously unimportant matters of detail. But that is by the by. It was for the GMC and the profession to make that good. I felt very positive about the idea of using the basic standard-setting model across the whole of UK healthcare. It was the model I was following for professional self-regulation, as I have explained. So, in terms of taking that agenda forward, the fact that the GMC modernisation could be put into the context of the wider national policy for health professions' regulation could only help in bringing about change.

The government was fortunate to have Liam Donaldson as CMO when the time came to put these proposals into action for he had well thought out ideas of how the various strands of quality in healthcare could be brought together into a single, coherent entity. He did a lot, behind the scenes, to help the government understand the practicalities of their quality agenda. I think it was also important that at such a critical time he and I found ourselves working together in two key roles, sharing very much the same vision. We had worked together before in the Northern Region. In 1991 we had published a comparative review of quality in healthcare in the UK and USA.[67] In this we had looked ahead to the new thinking which was beginning to integrate the public, professional, educational and managerial strands of quality in a way that had now become highly relevant.

The GMC

So this was the political and social context in which the profession and the GMC found itself in this critical period. The GMC was beginning to go under the microscope of public scrutiny in a way that had never happened before. It was thrust into the limelight, a situation for which it was ill-equipped to manage in terms of its professionalism in public relations. Investigative journalists got to work. In 1997 a *File on Four* programme took the GMC to task for its handling of doctors in private practice who were prescribing controlled drugs. In February 1998 there were three programmes in quick succession – a *Dispatches* programme on the GMC approach to erasure and restorations, a *World in Action* programme on drinking doctors and a *Newsnight* programme on why the GMC should not be trusted to look after patients' interests. Meanwhile, the GMC's Bristol hearing began on 13 October 1997 and was to draw huge press interest. Many will remember the images on television when, in February 1998, distraught parents demonstrated outside the GMC, placing a row of crosses on the pavement in memory of every child that had died.

Cultural change in the GMC

Between 1996 and 2001 the GMC went through substantial change in its own internal culture. The pace of change accelerated dramatically, as the timeline in Appendix C shows. This was partly driven from within the Council but it was hugely influenced by outside drivers as each big high-profile case, coming as they did in rapid succession, piled on the pressure. The GMC deserved to be criticised for matters for which it was clearly responsible. But it also became scapegoated by the government for deficiencies in the NHS which the government wished to minimise, and by the BMA which did not want to take responsibility for its own earlier lack of action on poor practice in what was after all professional self-regulation.

Some changes to the organisation were easy to make. They were structural and did not involve changes in behaviour. Finlay Scott, the Chief Executive, was able to make some early gains quickly. But most was far more difficult and fundamental. For example, a very real tension that underlay the GMC's logo and strapline 'protecting patients, guiding doctors' was only resolved decisively in favour of 'putting patients at the heart of everything we do' after the jolt of the Shipman case. Some medical members still interpret that unequivocal focus as diminishing concern for doctors and therefore difficult to accept.

Reform of Fitness to Practise

The reform of the GMC's Fitness to Practise procedures was by far the biggest, most difficult and most sensitive. Outside criticisms of slowness and lack of transparency helped to force change, but the real drivers were internal. It was virtually a case example itself of making cultural and organisational change. It is worth looking at more closely for that reason.

At my first Council meeting, in November 1995, I asked my colleagues to approve a major review of the Fitness to Practise procedures, especially the screening of complaints about doctors. Screening historically was a virtually enclosed process. The first real glimpse inside the box came through Isobel Allen's report[68] work for the Racial Equality Group, which looked into allegations of racial discrimination in the management of cases.* In her report of May 1996 she and her colleagues, highly expert and respected researchers, really laid bare for the first time – in evidential terms – just how completely inadequate the GMC screening systems were. They found that the GMC had neither a reliable database nor an effective way of tracking cases. It relied on the judgement of individual members – screeners – who made screening decisions at far too many points. The rule-bound processes were highly repetitive, each the cause of delay and possible error. In common with many public and semi-public organisations of the day, including the NHS itself, there were no operating standards, no mechanisms for monitoring, no audit and therefore no means of analysing aggregate data. So not surprisingly the GMC had no way of explaining to the outside world why it was making the decisions it did in individual cases. It could not even if it wanted to.

People who undertook screening were honest, straightforward members of the Council, both medical and lay. A general practitioner, Robin Steel, was the chief screener and had an excellent sense of

* During the six years that Isobel Allen's team looked into the question of racial discrimination in the Fitness to Practise procedures, many improvements were made. No overt racism was found. Nevertheless, there was a persistent unexplained difference between doctors who qualified overseas and UK-qualified doctors in their experience of the procedures.

judgement. It was not the people who were the problem, but the policies and systems themselves.

To help try to get to grips with this, Finlay and I asked the Audit Commission to do some external consulting work. Until 1995 I had been an Audit Commissioner. I knew their work well and had a high respect for their knowledge and experience of good process. At the same time we and the screeners for health commissioned the Department of Public Health Sciences at King's College, London and the Nuffield Institute for Health at the University of Leeds jointly to carry out an audit and evaluation of the GMC's health procedures in relation to handling 'sick' doctors.[69] The aim was to see if these were as good as rhetoric claimed them to be. The results were reassuring about the management of 'sick' doctors but less reassuring about the systems that underpinned the procedures, or the measures in place to make sure that sick doctors returning to practice were competent. These external reviews and audits, like Isobel Allen's work, were completely new to the GMC but were very much a part of the change process. They laid bare the problem without fudge. Painful though this was, they were the starting point for reconstruction.

This detailed work, at this stage, was fundamental in laying the foundations for the more radical changes that would have to come. The major overhaul of screening involved much painstaking and difficult work that called for a change of attitude as well as of practice in both the staff of the GMC and the screeners.

Keeping the pace, in September 1996 I proposed that the GMC establish a new Policy Committee charged with the oversight of policy development in Fitness to Practise and with responsibility for monitoring and reporting on results. The GMC had never had a mechanism for developing and synthesising policy in this, a vital component of its core business. It had been all *ad hoc*.

The new Committee was accepted warily – cultural suspicion again – and it took until May of the following year to get it established. There was considerable anxiety amongst both members and staff about the implementation of the performance monitoring function that I considered absolutely fundamental. The good news was that, once agreed, people began to see the benefits of the new way of working. The systematic work by that Committee, better data and new people who brought new skills and new perspectives began to make a difference. The Committee provided the mechanism and the focus of effort needed to rebuild Fitness to Practise machinery. The outcome, as I show later in Chapter 14, was a complete redesign from first principles. The implementation is not yet complete. But in the culture the outlook changed out of all recognition. Staff and members worked tremendously hard, and there was a good spirit. Data and transparency are still not what they should be, but that will change because now the will is there.

The value of lay involvement

Another example of cultural change was the attitude to lay involvement. That was changing positively in the early 1990s. But now we took a great stride forward in building on the benefits lay people brought. A critical mass of lay members, committed as they were to help the GMC get regulation right for doctors as well as patients, brought skills and expertise in their own right – skills in management, consumer affairs, politics, finance, the law, communications and so on. 'Layness' had a value in itself but these additional skills were value-added as they say. Lay members were appointed to chair major committees for the first time – Bob Nicholls to the Preliminary Proceedings Committee and Angela MacPherson to the new Interim Orders Committee.

The new performance assessors scrutinised the practice of doctors under the performance procedures and all were recruited by public advertisement from outside the GMC. A Council whose mindset had become attuned to the idea of medical–lay partnership saw it as natural that they would be trained together and work together in teams. That way of learning has now been extended to all working in Fitness to Practice activities. It has become the usual way of doing things.

Another example of joint working was with patient and consumer organisations on the development of revalidation, and later the final stages of the new Fitness to Practise procedures. In revalidation, we said that from the start the discussions on the development of methods to be used would be done on a partnership basis, with representatives of the doctors, the public, the employers and the GMC sitting down together. Each had to hear what others had to say. Most people considered it a successful and productive way of working. As a comment on that, I remember one of the consumer organisation people, frustrated at the DoH with the perception of tokenism so far as patient involvement was concerned, said 'Why don't you ask the GMC how to do it?' I knew then that we must be getting something right!

Concluding thought

Most people on the Council and those working for the Council felt bruised and battered by the sheer pressures and volume of work, and the pounding by the press, especially as the cases became public. But the drivers had their positive effect. It is a testimony to the Chief Executive and the majority of members and staff who wanted the GMC to move on that they succeeded in maintaining morale, and managed a major internal organisational and cultural change while leading change in the profession itself. Getting the profession to accept responsibility for doctors' continuing performance was the main issue for the next few years.

But first there was Bristol.

9

Bristol

Of all the high-profile failures in medicine that came to light in the 1990s, the events in paediatric cardiac surgery at the Bristol Royal Infirmary (BRI) were by far the most significant in dynamising change. They involved leading-edge 'high-tech' surgery. They were about infants and children. They involved a generalised systems failure as well as individual failings. They were about people trying to do the right things but clearly not always succeeding. They were not about evil people intent on deliberate harm.

The key facts

There were three key players at the heart of the GMC case. James Wisheart, trained at Queens University, Belfast, was a consultant in cardiac and thoracic surgery with the United Bristol Heathcare NHS Trust (UBHT). He had wider professional and management responsibilities that had included the Chair of the Hospital Medical Committee (1992–94), Associate Clinical Director of Cardiothoracic Surgery (October 1990–December 1993) and Medical Director from April 1992 until he retired in 1996. Between 1990 and 1993 he carried out 11 operations on babies for the correction of atrio ventricular septal defects (AVSD).* Five children died, a mortality rate of 45%. Over the next 18 months he carried out a further four operations on babies, all of whom died, so his overall mortality rate rose to 60%. At that point he stopped the operations on children.

Janardan Dhasmana was appointed as a consultant in cardio–thoracic surgery on 1 January 1986 in the unit led by Wisheart. His mortality rate for AVSD surgery was 10% – better than the national average and far better than Mr Wisheart's. His difficulties started when he began

---

* 'Hole in the heart'.

operating on babies – mainly children with Down's syndrome – with a congenital abnormality called 'transposition of the great vessels'. This was highly complex surgery that involved the reversing of the main arteries of the heart in babies who were born with them the wrong way round. Hence the term 'arterial switch operation'. Dhasmana carried out 38 arterial switch operations between 1988 and 1995 and 20 of the patients died. Nationally, the success rate ranged from 80%–90%.

John Roylance, a radiologist by background, was the first Chief Executive of the UBHT, which ran the Bristol Royal Infirmary. He was appointed in April 1991 after six years as District General Manager of the Bristol and Weston Health Authority. He was a well-known and respected radiologist. Although Chief Executive, he retained some clinical responsibilities in his own speciality.

The outline of the story is essentially this. Alarming statistics were already being reported in the Annual Report of the Bristol Unit for 1989–90. These appeared to show that deaths in operations on babies under one year of age were twice the British average. Stephen Bolsin was a young anaesthetist on the cardiac team through whose action as a whistle-blower the situation came to public notice. He had come recently to Bristol from the paediatric cardiac surgery unit at the Royal Brompton Hospital in London, that was doing similar procedures. He did his own calculations on figures available, on the basis of which he wrote a letter to Roylance expressing his concerns at the high mortality rate. He got no response but was referred to the then Director of Cardiac Services, James Wisheart, who was of course one of the two surgeons carrying out the operations. Dr Bolsin was rebuked for having written to Roylance.

As revealed later in the public inquiry, in 1992 the Royal College of Surgeons (RCS) reviewed and confirmed the data on fatalities and warned the Department of Health. Sir Terence English, President of the RCS at the time, found that the mortality at Bristol was disturbingly high. He communicated his concern to the DoH and added, in conjunction with the new President of the RCS, his own recommendation that Bristol should be de-designated as a cardiac surgery centre. This did not happen.

In 1994 Gianni Angelini, the newly appointed British Heart Foundation Professor of Cardiac Surgery at Bristol, carried out a new investigation at the request of the hospital Trust and the DoH. Angelini recommended that a new paediatric cardiac surgeon should be appointed, that the paediatric service should be moved to the children's hospital and that the complex neonatal switch operation should be halted. The first two recommendations were accepted by the Trust and were subsequently put into effect.

In 1994, the BRI had stopped performing arterial switch operations on neonates because of its bad record. However, in January 1995 a decision was made by the surgeons to carry out such an operation on the non-neonatal child, Joshua Loveday. The non-neonatal figures were thought to be acceptable. Mr Dhasmana was to carry out the operation. A special meeting of the clinical team was held the night before the operation to discuss it. This was chaired by Mr Wisheart. The parents were not told either of the BRI's high mortality record, or of the special meeting, or the fact that James Wisheart and John Roylance had already agreed that there should be an external review of the Unit's results. The DoH had raised its anxieties with the Trust. Nevertheless the surgeons decided to go ahead and Dr Roylance took no steps to stop them. The operation was carried out and Joshua died.

The GMC inquiry

On Thursday 28 March 1996 Channel 4 broadcast a special edition of *Dispatches*, a programme of their investigation into the record of cardiac surgery on infants and small children at Bristol. I did not see the programme. On Monday 1 April, an article in *The Times* by Lord Rees Mogg set out an alarming story. I and other GMC members saw that. The screener approved initial enquiries, although at that point no complaint had been received by the GMC. Shortly afterwards, in the first week in May, the GMC received a letter of complaint from Dr Bolsin. In the week beginning 17 June, the first complaint from a parent came in. The GMC's preliminary investigation began.

The GMC's inquiry proper started in mid-June 1996. It was to become the largest that the GMC had undertaken. The early inquiries ranged widely. In the course of these three doctors, two cardiologists and an anaesthetist, were sent what were called 'Chapter 15' letters. In these they were warned of possible proceedings against them. However, in the event the decision by the GMC Preliminary Proceedings Committee, advised by its investigating lawyers, was that there was sufficient evidence against the three doctors who were primarily involved – Mr Wisheart, Dr Roylance and Mr Dhasmana – to charge them with serious professional misconduct.

Whilst the GMC preparations were proceeding, there was considerable discussion in government about a public inquiry into all aspects of the events at Bristol. The Bristol parents wanted this wider examination to take place first before any GMC hearing. However, the government ultimately decided that the GMC inquiry should proceed first. In a written answer in the House of Commons, the Secretary of State Stephen Dorrell said that he believed that an inquiry would be necessary. However, since the GMC was already considering proceedings, he did not wish to prejudice its deliberations, so the public inquiry would not start till the GMC had completed its proceedings.

In October 1997, Mr and Mrs Stewart and other parents applied on behalf of their children to the High Court for leave to apply for judicial review of certain decisions relating to the forthcoming GMC hearing. This application, essentially seeking more information about the nature and scope of the evidence of the GMC inquiry with the intention of widening it, would have had the effect of delaying it. But the claim failed.

Early in the GMC investigation it was decided that as President I would chair the inquiry. It was normal practice for the President, if he was Chairman of the PCC, to do so, particularly in major cases. As a consequence of this decision, I was subject to the long-established GMC 'Chinese walls' procedure that precluded me from any knowledge of, or involvement in, the investigation and preparation of the case. As a result I then had no knowledge of what was happening other than what one could read in the newspapers as an ordinary citizen.

The GMC hearing began on 13 October 1997. It had been delayed for several months following an application from the defence who argued successfully before me that they had had insufficient time to prepare for the case. It proceeded, with some breaks, for a period of 74 sitting days in total, ending on 18 June 1998.

The charges

The purpose of a GMC conduct hearing is to consider allegations underlying a charge of serious professional misconduct. Unlike the later public inquiry, which was inquisitorial in nature, a GMC conduct hearing operates essentially like a criminal court. It is adversarial in nature. However, members of a panel or committee hearing a case are entitled to question witnesses and so play an important role. A case must be particularised in terms of specific allegations about specific events. Generalised opinion and unsubstantiated views, however many people share them, cannot be part of what are legal proceedings which may result in the loss of registration and therefore loss of livelihood and reputation for a doctor. This approach offered, as Rudolph Klein pointed out later, an inevitably powerful but selective searchlight because the charges in the case did not involve *all* the deaths at Bristol, only those cases where the evidence of potential SPM appeared to be strongest. The investigation was into the individual doctor's conduct.

At issue were 15 operations for the correction of AVSD in the case of

Mr Wisheart, and 30 arterial switch operations in the case of Mr Dhasmana.*

The nub of the GMC's case that lay behind the charges against the three doctors was this. Doctors have an ethical duty to practise within the limits of their professional competence. Moreover, they have an ethical duty to report poor practice where it may endanger patients. In a landmark case in 1994, an anaesthetist, Dr Dunn, was found guilty of SPM when he failed to act properly after being told by colleagues about the practice of a locum that was giving cause for grave concern. In the determination, which was widely publicised, the Conduct Committee said, 'Doctors who have reason to believe that a colleague's conduct or professional performance poses a danger to patients must act to ensure patient safety. Before taking action in such a situation doctors should do their best to establish the facts . . . . At all times patient safety must take precedence over all other concerns, including understandable reticence to bring a colleague's career into question.'

The crux of the charges against the surgeons was that they had failed to examine their own results critically enough, and to draw appropriate conclusions about the limits of their own performance. In particular they failed to stop operating – at least until the cause of the failures had been fully investigated and verified – when it should have been clear to them that colleagues had serious concerns about their results. It was this failure to stop and audit that led to avoidable death and damage to babies and small children. The charge against the Chief Executive, Dr Roylance, was that as a registered practitioner he failed to investigate or act on concerns when he was in a position and had a professional duty to do so.

Very experienced counsel represented the contributing parties.† The Committee sat with one of its most experienced legal assessors, Andrew Pugh, QC. The Legal Assessor's job is to ensure the fairness and impartiality of GMC proceedings, and to ensure that they are conducted within the requirements of the legal framework that the Committee has to follow. The Committee is an expert panel, not a jury – we had a mix of two experienced lay people and five doctors.‡

I have never witnessed such a detailed scrutiny of clinical cases before – the mixture of adversarial practice and inquiry left no clinical

---

* The numbers changed slightly during the course of the hearing as the charges were amended.
† Mr Duncan Matheson, QC and Mr Andrew Kennedy for Mr Wisheart, Miss Nicola Davies, QC and Mr Michael Partridge for Mr Dhasmana, Mr Robert Francis, QC and Ms Debra Powell for Dr Roylance. Roger Henderson, QC and Miss Rosalind Foster appeared for the GMC.
‡ The Committee in full: Sir Donald Irvine (chairing), Mr Rodney Yates and Ms Joanna White (lay), Professor Ken Hobbs (liver transplant surgeon), Dr Alum Khan (anaesthetist), Dr Jeremy Lee-Potter (pathologist) and Dr Fiona Pearsall (anaesthetist).

stones unturned, no clinical issues untested. The hearing involved the most rigorous scrutiny of individual cases operated on by the two surgeons. Many distinguished experts were called by all parties to contribute to that examination.

The hearing was emotionally highly charged both for the parents of the children and for the doctors whose registration was at stake as well as for all the others involved, including the panel itself. An example of that high emotion occurred just before Christmas. The defence lawyers had objected on several occasions to some members' questions, including my own. Then at this time I had told all parties out of courtesy that I had just found out that one of the cardiologists who was to be called by the GMC as an expert witness was very tangentially involved in the care of a family member. This was accepted by all, particularly as the matter concerned involved medical not surgical procedures – nothing remotely like the cases we were hearing described to us. A decision was made immediately by Counsel for the GMC not to call this witness. However, later Mr Francis on behalf of all the defence lawyers linked this issue to incisive questioning on my part. He invited the Committee to discharge itself, and/or for me to discharge myself, because of the alleged perception of bias on my part, and therefore prejudice by the whole Committee. The Committee, after hearing submissions from both sides and advice from the Legal Assessor, concluded that they were satisfied that there was no real or apparent bias. The case continued.

It is appropriate to add here that subsequently this decision by the Committee was one of the elements in the appeal by John Roylance to the Judicial Committee of the Privy Council against the GMC finding of SPM in his case. Their Lordships, in a detailed judgement, were 'not persuaded that either individually or collectively do the Chairman's questions disclose a biased approach . . . . They do not feel that he should have stood down from the inquiry nor that there was any unfairness in the conduct of the proceedings such as would warrant intervention'. The whole episode, however, was an indication of how high the stakes were.

The determination

James Wisheart and John Roylance were found guilty of SPM and were erased from the Medical Register. Janardan Dhasmana was also found guilty of SPM. However, in his case the Committee found mitigating circumstances. We noted that he 'took steps – albeit insufficient ones – to address the problems which you were facing. Furthermore, when you decided to operate on Joshua Loveday, Mr Wisheart and Dr Roylance had denied you crucial information'. Given this, the Committee directed that for a period of three years he should be required to stop undertaking paediatric cardiac surgery. That was the maximum period the Committee were allowed by law to impose. At the end of the three years there would be a resumed hearing.*

In the preamble to the determination (which is included in full as Appendix B), the Committee said:

> At the centre of this inquiry is the trust that patients place in their doctors. A parent placing a child in a doctor's care must have confidence that the doctor will put the child's best interests before any other. It is hard to imagine a situation in which trust is more essential. A doctor who fails to live up to that expectation will seriously undermine not only his or her relationship with that particular patient or parents, but the confidence of all patients in doctors.
>
> This Committee must and will take action where it appears that a doctor has betrayed that trust. At the same time, we have not allowed emotion to distract us from our duty, which is to consider a charge against each doctor. Our duty is to be fair and objective.

The Committee described the care taken to avoid judging the doctors with the benefit of hindsight. We said: 'We have kept firmly in mind that the most conscientious of doctors can, and do, make mistakes. People rightly expect high standards of doctors; but we must not judge doctors mercilessly according to the highest achievable performance. To do so would make medical practice impossible, and would be contrary to the interests of patients.'

The Committee added an important statement to the conclusion of its determination on the three doctors. It identified a number of general issues which arose during the course of its inquiry to do with the culture and practice of medicine, for which the three doctors were not held accountable but which the profession and others would have to address. They included:

- the need for clearly understood clinical standards
- how clinical competence and technical expertise are assessed and evaluated
- who carries the responsibility for team-based care

---

* There was, and the restriction on Mr Dhasmana was to continue for a further, fourth year. Then on 24 June 2002 the Committee decided that he had 'clearly demonstrated . . . that you will not carry out any procedures that you consider beyond your competence' and accepted Mr Dhasmana's statement that he would never again operate on children. They determined that there was 'no longer any necessity for the protection of members of the public for your registration to remain subject to any restrictions'.[70] The Committee complimented the excellent and original retraining programme devised for Mr Dhasmana by Mr Hilton, Mr Forty and Professor Dark at the Freeman Hospital, Newcastle upon Tyne. They commended it as a template for further retraining in a similar situation.

- the training of doctors in advanced procedures
- how to approach the so-called learning curve of doctors undertaking established procedures
- the reliability and validity of the data used to monitor doctors' personal performance
- the use of medical and clinical audit
- the appreciation of the importance of factors, other than purely clinical ones, that can affect clinical judgement, performance and outcomes
- the responsibility of a consultant to take appropriate actions in response to concerns about their performance
- the factors which appear to discourage openness and frankness about doctors' personal performance
- how doctors explain risks to patients
- the ways in which people concerned about patient safety can make their concerns known
- the need for doctors to take prompt action at an early stage where a colleague is in difficulty, in order to offer the best chance of avoiding damage to patients and the colleagues, and of putting things right.

Finally, the Committee noted the concern it had felt about the evidence suggesting institutional failures at the BRI and beyond. These were the systems issues that would need to be addressed urgently by the medical profession, the government and the NHS as well as the public inquiry that was to follow shortly.

Dr Roylance's appeal

Dr Roylance appealed to the Judicial Committee of the Privy Council against the Conduct Committee's decision. Their Lordships' judgement was delivered on 24 March 1999.[71] Besides the issue of alleged bias that I dealt with earlier, Dr Roylance sought to present a further argument about bias, levelled at the stage of the deliberations by the Committee on their final determination. Prior to the hearing of the full appeal he had sought from the Board an order to have the shorthand notes of the in camera deliberations of the Committee disclosed. That application was refused by their Lordships on 19 January 1999. However, he tendered an affidavit by Professor Peter Dunn, supporting an argument that there had been some unfairness in the course of the Committee's deliberations. Professor Dunn had written an article expressing a variety of concerns about the handling of the matter before the PCC. That had evidently prompted a telephone call from someone who was understood by Professor Dunn to have reliable information about what had passed during the in camera deliberations by the Committee. The identity of the informant was not disclosed to their Lordships. The affidavit set out some material that had been provided by this person to Professor Dunn.

Their Lordships accepted the affidavit *de bene esse** in order to understand more fully the substance of its contents, but having done so and heard argument they had come to a clear view that it should not be admitted as evidence in the appeal. In their judgement they noted:

> In the context of the making of any corporate judicial decision, the detail of discussion and the manner by which the decision is reached ought normally to remain confidential. In such a context it is essential for there to be opportunity for a frank exchange of views. In this way doubts and anxieties can be freely aired, opinions exchanged in the course of discussion with no necessary commitment to any final position, and eventually a conclusion reached, whether or not unanimously, with the confidence which can come from a mature, open and thorough consideration. It could only be in quite exceptional circumstances, if ever, that an inquiry could be permitted into such in camera discussions.

But they went further than that. They considered that not only was the applicant's application contrary to that general principle of confidentiality, but it was the more inappropriate in the particular context of the PCC. Unlike a jury, the Committee had the benefit of a Legal Assessor. Under the GMC's rules, the Assessor has an express duty not only to inform the Committee of an irregularity in the conduct of proceedings before them which comes to the Assessor's knowledge, but also to advise them of his/her own motion where it appears that there is a possibility of a mistake of law being made. That provision, their Lordships thought, appeared wide enough to cover improprieties in the process of discussion and determination of the issues before the Committee. Then there was the added point that under the rules parties are entitled to be informed of any advice tendered by the Legal Assessor after the Committee has begun to deliberate. The effect of that is that everyone has a right to know what advice on matters of law has been given. With that, and some further comment on the question of hearsay in connection with Professor Dunn's affidavit, they were 'not persuaded that the affidavit should be admitted nor that this area of the argument should be entertained'.

For the GMC, the testing of the argument about the confidentiality of in camera proceedings was of immense importance not simply in the context of this case, but more generally. The issues would arise from time to time in the Council in connection with other cases. But despite the

* Good for the present.

high emotion generated, the Law Lords supported the policy that confidentiality in that context is essential to a fair hearing.

Beyond the bias questions, Roylance questioned some of the findings of fact and therefore the reliability of the conclusions that could be drawn from them. Their Lordships did not find that any of the findings of fact by the Committee had been defective.

The most significant of elements of Roylance's appeal was that his actions as a manager should not be judged by the GMC as they did not involve his own clinical practice. The issue was about the extent to which a registered medical practitioner has a duty to protect patients. It was not disputed that Roylance undoubtedly had a duty to protect patients in his capacity as Chief Executive of the Trust, but it was not in that capacity that he came before the PCC of the GMC. His principal line of defence was that he owed no duty as a doctor. The problem was whether, given the fact of his being a registered medical practitioner in addition to his appointment as Chief Executive, he had any duties in respect of the former capacity in addition to his undoubted duties in respect of the latter. Dr Roylance's primary submission was therefore that during the period in question there had been no exercise by him of his professional judgement as a doctor.

Their Lordships pointed to the critical issue, namely, whether if there was misconduct, the misconduct was 'professional misconduct'. In their judgement the issue of the nature and extent of professional responsibility, and therefore of professional conduct, is fully explored. Dr Roylance, they held, was both a registered medical practitioner and Chief Executive of a hospital. In each capacity he had a duty of care for the safety and well-being of patients. As Chief Executive that duty arose out of his holding of that appointment. As a registered medical practitioner he had the general obligation to care for the sick. That duty did not disappear when he took the appointment but continued to co-exist with it. Their Lordships further observed that the GMC Committee had 'noted the particular circumstances of the history of growing anxiety, of the facts which they found of his knowledge of the concern, especially in the letter of 21 July 1994, and of his power to enquire and to intervene'. They (the GMC panel) affirm that as a registered medical practitioner the appellant had a duty to act to protect patients from harm. The GMC Committee had said in their determination that:

> Your own evidence demonstrates that you chose, over a long period, to ignore the concerns which were being brought to your attention, preferring to leave these matters to the consultants concerned. Yet, faced with information suggesting that children were being placed unnecessarily at risk, you took no steps to establish the truth. You knew that your Medical Director was at the centre of many of these

concerns, yet you took no steps to obtain impartial advice from appropriate specialists.

Their Lordships concluded that 'essentially it was the appellant's own belief that his being a registered practitioner was irrelevant that was the flaw in his defence'. Roylance's appeal on this count was not allowed. This conclusion is very important. It underlined the fact that any doctor, in accepting the privileges of registration with the GMC, is obligated to discharge the duties that go with them. That judgement underscored the more explicit link subsequently established between professional standards and their observance even by doctors not themselves engaged in clinical practice.

So on all points the appeal was dismissed.

Immediate reactions

At the conclusion of the GMC inquiry feelings amongst the parents were running high. There was much public anger and serious anxiety in the profession. There was a huge number of press and television cameras outside the GMC headquarters in Hallam Street in London. People were held back by railings, and the police were everywhere trying to enable the defendants to get out safely in the face of the hostile crowds. Two impressions above all stand out for me from those moments. One was my memory of one of the distraught parents, Mrs Willis, who was in the public gallery of the hearing chamber as I was finishing reading the determination, and broke the silence to shout that the GMC proceedings had been a 'charade'. On the other hand there was another parent who I did not know who said to me as I was leaving the building 'How dare you strike off Mr Wisheart – he is such a fine surgeon'. As I walked outside three others standing together simply said 'thank you'. The passionate feelings of these parents, reflecting completely different personal experiences, seemed to epitomise the tragedy of Bristol.

In the prevailing atmosphere the decision of the Committee not to strike off Janardan Dhasmana, although finding him guilty of SPM, was likely to be the most challenging. Many people – to some extent understandably – wanted blood. In the event the early news broadcasts were quite neutral in their reporting of the GMC's decision. However the response from other quarters was swift, not least from Frank Dobson, the Secretary of State for Health. Interviewed later that night on *Newsnight*, he made it clear that he thought that the GMC should have struck Mr Dhasmana off the register. He said, 'I think under the circumstances and what I know of the evidence, if they struck off the two doctors, they should have struck off all three.' He was clearly very angry. He may have felt as he did in his private capacity as an individual who was not privy to all the facts. However, as Secretary of State for Health and legally the employer of the doctors concerned, he should not have expressed his feelings publicly without having heard any part of the evidence or being party to the discussions and deliberations.

Although I liked and respected Frank Dobson, I was angry with him about what I felt was a completely inappropriate and inflammatory response, so I made a point of going to see him shortly afterwards and we had, as they say, a frank exchange of views. I told him that I felt he had gone beyond his responsibilities as Secretary of State in undermining what had been a properly constituted, careful and fair inquiry. He for his part told me how disappointed he was that the new-look GMC that he thought was in the making could come to such a decision. We then had what I felt was a constructive lengthy discussion about the next steps. I supported his quality agenda. Equally he was, I know, strongly supportive of what I was trying to do with the GMC.

It was Richard Smith's editorial in the *BMJ*[2] that seemed to capture the reactions of the medical profession best. 'The Bristol case', he said, 'will probably prove to be much more important to the future of healthcare in Britain than the reforms suggested in the White Papers . . . . The Bristol case is a once in a lifetime drama that has held the attention of doctors and patients in a way that a White Paper can never hope to match.'

He (and Richard Horton, Editor of the *Lancet*) castigated Frank Dobson for what he described as a 'serious mistake' on *Newsnight*. But he also took the wider view. Regulation was not just about the GMC. In particular, he emphasised the importance of local self-regulation as the most likely means of influencing doctors' behaviour on a day-to-day basis.

Horton, in two thoughtful leaders, concentrated on the professional issues raised at the end of the determination. He was strongly supportive of the GMC's strategy for modernising professional regulation, although, he noted, 'Their efforts have been largely ignored by the public, and most doctors are probably unaware of the profound implications that follow from the GMC strategy.'[78]

Hospital Doctor, the weekly newspaper for doctors working in hospitals, gave the GMC 'full marks for a bold judgement'. Noting that the GMC had just come through one of the biggest tests in its 140-year history, it had emerged with credit, unlike many others involved. It was particularly pleased that the panel had stood firm 'against massive public pressure, not to mention Health Secretary Frank Dobson'. The public, it noted, had wanted Mr Dhasmana's head, but it considered that it would have been a travesty if he had been struck off: 'Given the circumstances, the fact that the Committee did not sacrifice Dhasmana to protect itself, is all the more impressive.'

Professor Rudolph Klein, in an excellent analytical paper[72] on the substance of Bristol and the GMC inquiry, explored many of the wider cultural issues for the profession. He focused particularly on the need for more effective local regulation and the difficult question of collective responsibility and accountability in clinical teams. On the inquiry itself, he commented on its limitations, the patchy glimpses it gave of the wider picture, but he commended the rigour of the process as actually operated by the GMC within the statutory limits governing its remit and procedures.

But as to public confidence in the GMC, he felt that the inquiry provided 'one clear, emphatic and welcome answer. If there were any doubts about the GMC's commitment to its contract with the public, about its determination to demonstrate the profession's collective acceptance of responsibility for maintaining competence in practice, they have been dispelled. And that should send a powerful message both to the profession itself and to the public.'

Parents' groups

The events at Bristol led the parents involved to form the Bristol Parents' Action Group. This provided a base for mutual support and help, and was a powerful mechanism through which the parents could promote their case at every level in the system. They were well connected with the press. They became the focal point for the parents' views of what was needed by way of reform. I believe that overall they were an immense force for good because they, by their very existence and the assertive reasonableness of their approach, made it compellingly clear to all that the voice of the patient had to be heard and heeded.

Other groups incidentally sprung up at about the same time. The women damaged by Rodney Ledward and by Richard Neale formed their own group. The relatives of Harold Shipman's victims did likewise. And the parents at the Liverpool Children's Hospital at Alder Hey became a very powerful focus for articulating and taking action as they thought appropriate following the retained body parts scandal around Professor Van Veltzen.

All the groups had excellent cross-links and communications. Thus was born a new dimension in healthcare – the articulate, organised and highly motivated force driven by the victims of medical accidents.

The Kennedy Report

The public inquiry[1] chaired by Professor (now Sir) Ian Kennedy was conducted between October 1998 and July 2001. There were two phases, one focusing on events at Bristol, the other on the future. The inquiry was huge. On Bristol alone, written evidence was received from 577 witnesses, including 238 parents. The medical records of over 1800 children were examined. The inquiry was very skilfully conducted. In particular, the inquiry team went out of its way to make sure that the parents were able to tell their story, and to be fully involved throughout.

The essential findings were as follows. In respect of the paediatric cardiac surgical services at Bristol, the inquiry found that in general terms healthcare professionals working at Bristol were caught up in a combination of circumstances 'which owed as much to the general failings in the NHS at the time'. Nevertheless there were failures by individuals on occasions in the care of sick children. There were problems with a split site for the provision of paediatric open-heart surgery, no dedicated paediatric intensive-care beds, no full-time paediatric cardiac surgeon and too few trained nurses. There were issues involving 'a club culture', an imbalance of power with too much control in the hands of too few people. There was a lack of means for assessing the quality of care, and no standards against which to evaluate performance. The inquiry concluded that there was confusion throughout the NHS as to where responsibility lay for performance monitoring. Overall, Kennedy concluded this 'flawed' system at Bristol led to around one-third of all the children who underwent open-heart surgery receiving less than adequate care. The inquiry commissioned an independent assessment of the quality of the paediatric cardiac services at Bristol. The experts' principal finding was that 'the single most compelling aspect of the data is the magnitude of the discrepancy between the outcomes observed at Bristol and elsewhere. For children undergoing open heart surgery between 1988 and 1994, the observed mortality rate at Bristol was roughly double that observed elsewhere in five out of seven years.' Kennedy's recommendations are referred to in Chapter 15 as they complemented and reinforced the changes the government and the medical profession had already made to the system.

The inquiry made detailed criticisms of James Wisheart as a clinician and a medical director. John Roylance was subject to criticism as a manager. Janardan Dhasmana was only lightly criticised, being seen more as a victim of the system than as a cause in his own right.

The implications and impact of Bristol are told in the rest of this book. For myself, the seven months of the GMC hearing itself were the most taxing and demanding of my professional life.

Concluding comment

I have only one comment to add. Some in my profession have said that the three Bristol doctors were scapegoated by the GMC. I do not accept that criticism. As both the GMC and Kennedy inquiries showed, there was a range of professional and institutional failures. Both found personal culpability, albeit from different perspectives. The distinction between individual and wider systems responsibilities was made quite clear in the determination by the GMC panel hearing the case (*see* Appendix B). Each doctor had the right of appeal to the Privy Council against the decision in his case. Dr Roylance chose to exercise that right, and their Lordships found against him.

This brings me to a more general point. There is a view, gaining some currency these days in the medical profession, that in the event of medical tragedies, one should 'blame the system' rather than point to individuals. This is coupled with the altogether wider movement for a 'no-blame' culture. I think the term 'no blame' is actually unhelpful. It can become so easily associated with the abrogation of responsibility. It might be better to seek a 'fair culture' that attributes responsibility appropriately. In this, if there have been personal failings they have to be addressed. Individual doctors have to accept responsibility where it falls to them, just as they accept the accolades. Public trust depends on doctors exercising their skills and experience to the best of their ability and within their competence. Identifying problems with – and improving – the systems will only work if individuals are open about, and accept their responsibility for, their part in any error or failure. People run systems, they do not run themselves. The bottom line is doctors' individual accountability. We should expect no less.

Part 4
Achieving the change:
the real story

10

Regular checks for doctors: revalidation is born

As the GMC Bristol hearing was nearing its end, minds on all sides were turning to what would happen next. The government was putting the final touches to its new White Paper on quality in the new NHS that we understood they planned to launch around the time the case ended.

At the May GMC meeting of Council, Cyril Chantler and his colleagues on the Standards Committee had cleared the latest edition of *Good Medical Practice*,[73] which in its introduction now linked standards explicitly with registration. It was to be launched before the hearing ended together with a new booklet, *Maintaining Good Medical Practice*,[74] that set out the principles of internal clinical governance in clinical teams, and told doctors explicitly what to do, step by step, when there were doubts about a colleague's practice. All in all there had been much good work done on these elements of our programme.

However, the GMC was having difficulty in getting doctors (and the NHS) to take *Good Medical Practice* as seriously as we thought necessary. Studies carried out[75,76] by the GMC in 1997–98 showed variable awareness by doctors of *Duties of a Doctor* and *Good Medical Practice*. Variations in attitude were recorded. For example, senior NHS professionals were reluctant to consider poor consultation skills in the same critical light as they did persistently poor technical practice. Doubts therefore remained about whether the regular annual appraisal of doctors that the government was planning would be sufficient to change the culture and make medicine more secure overall. These doubts raised the issue of the recertification of doctors once again. In an informal meeting with Frank Dobson and Alan Milburn on 31 March 1998, my colleagues and I had expressed our doubts about the usefulness of the Specialist Register in its current form. We suggested that we should be considering whether a doctor's continued entry on the Specialist Register might be conditional upon 'revalidation' at intervals. We were all aware of the public expectation that medical regulation should include measures to assure patients that consultants and general practitioners continue to perform effectively throughout their working lives.

On Tuesday 16 June 1998, in the interval between the announcement of the findings of fact in the Bristol case (and the huge press coverage that followed) and the announcement of the final determination, I went with Finlay Scott to an informal dinner at the Academy of Medical Royal Colleges. I noted in my diary that 'it may be that it turned into one of those defining points'. I was now quite clear that a response to Bristol from the GMC and the profession would have to address head on – and promptly – this issue of the ongoing competence of doctors. That meant re-certification. I went with our agenda for the development of our professionalism and medical regulation and how this should be shaped to take account of the lessons of Bristol. I outlined the GMC's thinking and the further development of the relationship we would be looking for in future with the Colleges. This discussion was serious and wide-ranging, reflecting the uncertainties of the time.

The Colleges were the repositories of standards in their specialities, and they would need to indicate good performance in their members and possibly all those on the Specialist Register. We emphasised the need to strengthen the links with specialist societies and associations because of their expertise in their clinical subjects.

The 'Dear Roddy' letter

Following that meeting and further internal discussion, I wrote on 30 June 1998 to the Academy what has now become known as the 'Dear Roddy' letter. It was this letter that effectively fired the starting gun for revalidation. I recalled the discussion on 16 June in which we had gone over the GMC's basic strategy for securing and maintaining good medical practice:

- clear general and specific standards
- effective local, medical regulation based on quality-assured practice – clinical governance
- effective local and central arrangements for dealing with poor practice.

I recalled how, in the course of our conversation, we had spoken about the place of the Specialist Register within this general approach, its use today, and the gap between its current function and wider public perception.

I emphasised the clear public expectation that medical regulation should include measures to assure patients that consultants, and general practitioners, continue to perform effectively throughout their working lives. At the same time I reflected our questioning of the usefulness of the Specialist Register in its current form:

> Can it be sufficient, for example, that a doctor, once admitted to the Specialist Register, remains on it indefinitely, subject only to remaining on the Medical Register itself? Alternatively, what assurance does the Specialist Register offer patients and employers other than that, at a point in time, the doctor, perhaps many years before, gained a Certificate of Completion of Specialist Training, or held a consultant appointment? The answer is none, in the present form. The GMC is accountable for the fitness for purpose, and the effectiveness, of the Specialist Register. I do not believe that we can reconcile that accountability with its present limitations . . . One obvious possibility would be to make a doctor's continued entry on the Specialist Register conditional upon revalidation at, say, five-year intervals.

I wrote to the BMA and heads of medical schools in similar terms. I knew that the letter, when made public, as it would be, gave a statement undermining the current reliability of the Register from which there could be no retreat. But to know that the Register was unreliable and not act would have been irresponsible, whatever the medico-political consequences might be.

To my relief the Academy responded promptly and positively, as did the leaders of the BMA and the heads of medical schools. To maintain the momentum, and indeed to commit ourselves openly and publicly so that there would be no second thoughts, I proposed a meeting with all the profession's leaders to be held at the GMC on 27 August. The purpose was to talk about the revalidation of registration.

At that time there was a flurry of informal discussions with some Council members and professional leaders. Then I sent the letter of invitation to set the agenda and in which I set out the proposal in as positive terms as possible. These were that the purpose of revalidation would be to enable consultants and principals in general practice to confirm and demonstrate the quality of their professionalism to the outside world. Ideally, each speciality would assume ownership of the detailed arrangements and methods for its field of practice, as happens in the steps leading to the certification of specialist training and vocational training for general practice already. The methods used should reflect doctors' continuing professional development and performance at work, and should use existing data wherever possible.

These external reviews could be complemented by the information about the doctor's performance that should become available routinely in future within clinical teams, as a result of local medical regulation and clinical governance. 'Then', I said, 'one can begin to see how well-founded arrangements could evolve without making excessive new demands on doctors who are already stretched.'

As part of the preparation for this important meeting the President's Advisory Committee met on 30 July 1998. We discussed how best to get *Good Medical Practice* and *Maintaining Good Medical Practice* into the minds not only of everyone on the Medical Register, but also all the chairpeople and chief executives of health authorities, trusts and health boards. We felt: 'No one should be under any illusion: what is expected of a doctor is what is set out in *Good Medical Practice*, and the basis of quality-assured practice in every clinical directorate, every clinical unit, should include standard setting, audit and appraisal.'

Julia Neuberger, a lay member, had met the Tory and Liberal Democrat shadow teams at the King's Fund within the past few days. There had been a very strong message that they – the politicians – were ready to pick a fight with the medical profession. Ergo the need for fast action by the GMC and the profession. This view was reinforced by the recent lunch Finlay Scott and I had had with Ann Widdecombe, the then shadow Secretary of State for Health. She started off the conversation by saying 'One more like that [Bristol] and you can say goodbye to self-regulation'. We could all sense that there was a strong tide running against the profession and that the whole profession was seen as having let patients down in one way or another. The angst was not at that stage primarily focused on the GMC, but rather on the Colleges, largely because of their close involvement in Bristol through the Royal College of Surgeons. Also I told the PAC of my recent meeting with officers of the Society of Cardiothoracic Surgeons of Great Britain and Ireland, post Bristol, in which they had been very thoughtful, constructive and determined. There had been other meetings with George Alberti, President of the RCP, together with nephrologists, diabetologists and specialists in respiratory medicine, about the interesting methods of peer review that they were developing.

Lastly, and indicative of the public and government mood, we reflected on a discussion by the 'Top Nine',* the leaders of the profession, who had decided that, post Bristol, there should be some kind of public statement which would demonstrate a unified profession. I had reservations about making such a statement because I was dubious about what

* These were the Heads of the following medical institutions: General Medical Council, BMA GP and specialist committees, Council of Deans, Joint Consultants' Committee, Postgraduate Deans, Academy of Royal Medical Colleges, STA and JCPTGP.

rhetoric would achieve. The public was looking for action from the medical profession, not more promises. Nevertheless a statement was produced by the Joint Consultants' Committee, the BMA and others. In the event it had precisely the opposite effect of that intended. To the outside world it was perceived as defensive, as an expression of hope rather than a statement of substance. One commentator said, 'Who do the Top Nine think they are?' and 'Why are they all male and white?' – a clear indication of the kind of mood around.

In the discussion on revalidation there were two main strands in the PAC's thinking at that point. One was the need to make full use of the data on a doctor's performance that should flow from clinical governance and the annual appraisal the government planned for all NHS doctors. The second was that there would need to be some kind of external review of a doctor's practice. The basis would vary from speciality to speciality, but in general the external peer review the general practice trainers were using and the physicians and surgeons were exploring was forming the background to the thinking.

There was considerable discussion on the need for public involvement in the process of developing revalidation as well as engaging the profession. This was emphasised particularly by the lay members but the medical members needed no persuading. There was also the need for really effective communications with Council members from whom there were already hints of grumbles about lack of consultation, especially from those who were opposing revalidation. There were strong feelings from some – from those who supported revalidation as well as those who did not – that I should have consulted the Council first at the coming November meeting rather than go to the leaders of the profession in August. Others were strongly supportive of the rapid response. We all agreed on the need for good communication, and consequently I wrote to all Council members setting out the position.

The critical meeting: 27 August 1998

This was such an important meeting in reflecting where the leaders of the profession stood at that time that it is worth recalling in some detail.* I gave a very short introduction – uncharacteristically short for me! The meeting had before it an equally short paper that was based on the two letters that had gone to the Academy and the BMA.

I explained that I sought this early meeting with the leaders of the profession because I felt it was important to find out what they thought about the revalidation proposal, in private, before the matter was aired in

* The summary is from a transcript of the meeting.

the GMC Council meeting in public. I hoped everyone would agree that presenting a picture at this initial stage of a profession in disarray, or indecisive on a measure now clearly central to public safety, would be about the worst possible signal we could give to the outside world.

Ian Bogle, now Chairman of the BMA, began the discussion by saying that he accepted the principle of having a robust and demonstrable means of assuring the public and the profession, probably through a process of periodic revalidation. He agreed about the need for speed. He reminded the meeting of recent examples of how the profession, particularly in general practice, had attempted to get to grips with the principle of re-certification before – for instance in the selection of training general practices. But the problem had been that the trainers were largely self-selected and self-motivated with an interest in quality and education already. He was firm that we must all be clear about how to put the principle used with them into practice in order for it to apply to all doctors on the Medical Register.

Jim Johnson, who was then Chairman of the BMA Central Consultants' and Specialists' Committee (CCSC), noted that they had just had a debate in the BMA Council that was supportive of the principle, but that the details would be very important. He made the point: 'If it [revalidation] is for every speciality and it will be at regular intervals and it will continue forever, then the DoH will have to be involved in it and sign up to it. We have not really started on that yet. For us that is the *sine qua non.*'

There were of course some immediately important consequential issues such as how it would affect retired people on the Register, the writing of medical reports by non-practising doctors and so on.

Dr Andrew Porter, speaking as a junior doctor, said that revalidation represented 'quite an opportunity for junior doctors'. He had some reservations about the idea, particularly that 'for the rest of our careers we will spend time revalidating each other and ourselves'. However, he saw the potential for replacing some of the forms of assessment used in specialist training at the moment, and he made a plea for modernising specialist training through, for example, having an exit examination for all specialities.

Several speakers emphasised their view that examinations as a form of revalidation would be counter-productive. They would be short term and inhibit the culture of continuing professional development. Colin Smith (BMA), for example, favoured appraisal and performance review and had done so for many years. His approach to this was very much on the basis of personal skills development and enhancement through audit and peer review.

Mac Armstrong, who was then Secretary of the BMA, suggested that it would be a good idea to go outside of the profession to get some fresh ideas about the mechanics of revalidation. He noted the contractual issues that would have to be dealt with and that we would need to 'trust each other to get them sorted out'.

Surendra Kumar (Chairman of the Overseas Doctors' Association) spoke positively from the point of view of the overseas-qualified doctors. He went beyond the principle to consider: 'How are we to sell it? It will not be easy, but I believe that at the end responsibility lies with those sitting round this table to go out and do it.'

Brian Keithley, again from general practice, accepted the principle and alluded to the vacuum on quality that he thought existed at the moment. He referred to a meeting he had attended at the DoH on clinical governance: 'I do not think that the Department had any clear idea on how to assess the quality of clinical governance in an independent contractor profession.' His preference for a professional initiative was clear: 'I would rather have something rooted in professional self-regulation than a government-led inspectorate, which seems to be heralded by some of the documents and the centralist approach taken so far.' He referred, as many other speakers had done, to the need for proper resourcing to get the project under way properly.

Cyril Chantler, a dean of medicine and a paediatrician, was there for the Council of Heads of Medical Schools. He was very clear that 'we must decide whether we accept the notion that to be on the Medical Register implies that the individual is competent. I am sure that that is what the British public assumes, but it is not always the reality. It is very important that we develop ways to demonstrate that.' He went on to emphasise that assessing the individual would be insufficient; there is the matter of the clinical team in which individuals participate: 'Part of the appraisal system must be: how good is that individual at playing a part in the team?'

John Temple, who spoke for the postgraduate deans welcomed the principle, but he cautioned that we must 'be very careful that we do not step into the area of fairly major duplication of effort, simply because the whole thrust of government policy is making sure that at a local level there are good systems in place to guarantee to everyone that those who deliver care are capable.' He wanted to be absolutely sure that we put in place 'a system that is complementary and not separate from that'. So he was not concerned with the principle but very concerned about the process.

Roddy MacSween, Chairman of the Academy of Medical Royal Colleges, said that the message that had emerged from discussions was that the Academy would support the process of revalidation and would encourage the GMC to proceed along this route. He foresaw the Academy having a role in producing an overall background against which individual colleges could work on the detail. He saw revalidation becoming a means of bringing people together, leading to the embedding of peer review on a day-to-day basis: 'A formative and summative assessment would be part of professional life from the time one is a medical student until one retires.'

George Alberti (Academy), whilst agreeing with the principle, spoke against examinations which he said 'would be a disaster'.

Denis Pereira Gray (Academy), identified four principles that had been identified, namely, that the system should be founded on evidence, that it should be nationally consistent, that it should be performance based, and that it should be practice-based and practice-sensitive. He cited the work done on *Fellowship by Assessment* in the RCGP in particular, as an example of what could be done.

Leo Strunin, also for the Academy, spoke for the anaesthetists who had already tried to put together a document on good medical practice for anaesthetists and who of course had done a lot of the preparatory work on the assessment of anaesthetists' performance for the GMC performance procedures. Being an anaesthetist, with so much of the work team based, he drew attention to the fact that many of the things that had become high profile were not the failures of individual doctors but rather of systems.

The meeting went on to discuss many of the practicalities and the anxieties that would have to be handled. However, the key message that I took away was just how positive and unanimous the profession's leaders were in recognising that an appropriate and bold response was the right way forward.

I felt both relieved and encouraged by the general reactions. But we all knew that we had been expressing essentially our own personal views. No one was under any illusion – the journey would be a difficult one as the wider the profession became involved. And as many said 'the devil would be in the detail'.

I wrote in my diary at the end of that day:

> This should mean a good head of steam to take the matters forward when [the] various councils and committees meet in September/ October. By then also I hope to have overcome some of the mutterings from our own Council members that I have jumped the gun on this. All the time I am aware that the new NHS bill will be into the public domain in October and I am very anxious that the profession has positioned itself properly by then on what should be seen as a very positive step to strengthen medical accountability.

Yet I was clear in my own mind that, even now, the consensus achieved would not have been possible without the state of shock induced in the profession by the revelations at Bristol and, especially, the power of the public's response.

Twenty-two years had passed since the profession, through the Alment Committee, had first addressed the question of continuing fitness to practise and recertification (*see* Chapter 5).

11

Revalidation: the first debates

In that late summer, extensive discussions centred on the new regulatory agenda. There were two important meetings between representatives of the GMC and the NHS Executive. The first, in the immediate aftermath of my meeting with Frank Dobson, had been planned for another purpose, but Ken Calman and I adapted it for a post-mortem on Bristol. Alan Langlands, the Chief Executive of the NHS and Yvonne Moores, the CNO of England were there. They reflected serious anxieties as to whether the GMC was prepared to go far enough with reform. As we understood it, ministerial attitudes to the GMC were hardening because of the decision not to strike off Janardan Dhasmana. The second meeting, on 20 October, was about our response to the White Paper on quality. There was clear common ground on clinical governance, and concern on both sides about the poor alignment between the GMC and NHS complaints procedures.

In the run-up to the Council meeting there was extensive discussion as resistance to the idea of revalidation built up outside from some sectors of the profession, but there was also open support. For example, on Thursday 22 October the Senate of Surgery, comprising all the surgical colleges, held a press conference on their response to Bristol in which they were strong on their decision to adopt revalidation. The Academy of Medical Royal Colleges had come out positively, and I knew that Ian Bogle hoped that the BMA would do likewise. And later, on 28 October, at a meeting of the profession's leaders with Frank Dobson and his team, I noted in my diary that the Colleges were solid. Ian Bogle and John Chisholm, both from the BMA and both general practitioners, spoke strongly and positively about it. The doubts, I noted, came from Peter Hawker and Jim Johnson, also from the BMA and consultants.

The shadow of Rodney Ledward

In this period of change and uncertainty, we now had the next of the 'case drivers'.

Rodney Ledward was a consultant gynaecologist and obstetrician at the South Kent Hospitals NHS Trust. He also operated on gynaecological patients privately. Indeed, his negligent practice first came to public notice after an incident in January 1996 involving a private patient, in which he perforated her bladder during a hysterectomy at St Saviour's Hospital. Despite the appearance of blood in her urine, Ledward ordered a test and left the hospital and switched off his mobile phone. As the patient's condition deteriorated, hospital staff made urgent attempts to contact him without success. She was later admitted to hospital for further emergency surgery. The Medical Director of the hospital was so concerned that Ledward was suspended four days later.

At the beginning of February 1996 Ledward had been suspended by the Trust and at the end of 1996, after an inquiry by the Trust and disciplinary proceedings, he was summarily dismissed by the Trust from his post. The internal Trust inquiry examined 150 operations carried out by Ledward and found a third had resulted in serious complications with 12 showing evidence of incompetence. Ledward, as the later Committee of Inquiry[77] was told, was seen as 'a breath of fresh air' in the Department of Obstetrics and Gynaecology and he came with excellent recommendations and a high professional standing. He was acknowledged to have a good academic reputation and was very enthusiastic. One of his former patients described him as 'very dashing – quite the *Women's Weekly* hero'. He was flamboyant, a colourful character with bow tie, black jacket and pinstripe trousers and a liking for fast cars. Ledward prided himself on being known as 'the fastest gynaecologist in the South East'. His flamboyance and self-confidence verged on the arrogant. He would visit his patients in jodhpurs on a Sunday morning.

Ledward was referred to the GMC, which, following further extensive investigations, heard allegations about 14 cases. Rodney Ledward's problems with his practice, that is, an exceptionally high complication rate, were evident almost from the time of his first appointment. On 30 September 1998 he was struck off the Medical Register for providing a standard of care that the PCC said was 'lamentably below that which the public requires and which the medical profession expects of its members'.

The press reactions were devastating. This was another blow to the profession. The issue, in terms of public safety, was why it had taken so long for action to be taken by Ledward's employers, when it was known that a number of his consultant colleagues, and local general practitioners and nurses, were bringing forward their concerns. For me Ledward simply reinforced my view that good clinical governance underpinned by revalidation was a 'must.' Prevention had to be better than acting after the event.

The Council debates but fails to decide

The Council debated revalidation for the first time on Wednesday 4 November 1998.[78] As a general point, at the outset, everyone present was signed up to the government's new proposals for clinical governance, including clinical auditing, CPD and annual appraisal. This would be the first time that doctors would experience appraisal in their NHS practice, although those with university appointments were used to it in connection with their academic work. So one issue was what would revalidation add?

It was a lively occasion and the public were able to hear it all. The general tenor of the debate and the mood was good but anxious, with pros and cons being expressed and explored by many speakers. It was Ed Borman, a member of the BMA Hospital Consultants and Specialists Committee (HCSC), who led the argument against. Accepting all the reasons for doctors keeping up to date, and showing that they do, Dr Borman nevertheless objected to what he called the 'hard' linkage which would mean that a doctor who did not sustain their performance could be taken off the Register and so be unemployable. To achieve such a linkage, he argued there 'would have to be a valid assessment of performance and . . . legally defensible standards of proof of that'. He saw methodological difficulties with that. He concluded: 'I feel that linkage to the Register is inappropriate; it is open to legal challenge; it would be difficult to defend on the basis of standard of proof, and it is unnecessary in the light of current advances – which themselves will ensure that we doctors provide safe care for our patients.' Others supported his line of argument. Fiona Pearsall, an anaesthetist, referred to the proposals as 'ill-conceived and poorly defined.' Jim Appleyard, then also the BMA Treasurer, asked for the evidence that revalidation would add anything, and cited American experience. He referred also to a 'climate of fear' in the profession.

Thereafter the debate ebbed and flowed. The final turning point came with the contribution by the radiologist, Gill Markham. She entirely supported the view that doctors must be up to date and show their fitness to practise but – and it was a big but – she thought that this could all be done by contract and clinical governance. She argued persuasively that with so much change, at this stage, the profession did not need more.

The government was introducing clinical governance with appraisal part of it for doctors in any case. Wait and see how clinical governance worked out.

This argument was almost immediately picked up by no less than David Carter, the CMO for Scotland. He strongly allied himself with Gill's position and suggested that the GMC was 'in danger of creating a monster', with one half of the profession policing the other. It was, I felt and recorded at the time, unhelpful and surprising, particularly from someone so committed to professional standards. He opened the way – wittingly or unwittingly – for the opponents of revalidation and the genuine doubters to pick up his theme. Many Council members were very unsettled by this, including those who were well disposed to the idea. They now seemed to be unsure as to where the policy line would flow between the managerial proposals of government and our own professional regulatory ideas.*

Julia Neuberger (lay member) really put her finger on a problem of understanding. Accepting the argument put by Gill Markham and David Carter, she said that nevertheless for her the nub was that 'The GMC, the registration body, says these people are doctors; but does it continue to keep people on the Register when they have really no idea whether they are any good or not?' She believed it was critical, therefore, that the GMC make the case that registration means a demonstration of fitness to practise, is nationwide and has proper lay involvement.

Given the uncertainties, it was another lay member, Bob Winter, who proposed that the issue be left on the table. By unanimous vote, the Council decided that 'specialists and general practitioners must be able to demonstrate – on a regular basis – that they are keeping themselves up to date and remain fit to practise in their chosen field'. With only one vote against, we established a steering group so that further work could begin in preparation for a full preliminary debate on the issues of implementation (of revalidation) at the forthcoming February 1999 Conference. And on the motion of Bob Winter, who was genuinely undecided on the basis of the argument so far, the Council decided to leave on the table until the next meeting the principle of linkage with registration. Forty-nine voted for waiting, 38 were against and one abstained.

I felt keenly disappointed. I was dismayed that on the face of it we had achieved a really unsatisfactory outcome. It did not present the picture of a decisive profession that I had hoped we would see. Furthermore, Dr Ali (Council member) had earlier pointed to the inconsistency that 'we voted unanimously this morning to protect the power of the GMC in

* Such was my concern about the implication of what David Carter had said that I spoke to him next day. There was clearly much more divergence in government thinking at that stage between Scotland and England. Any misconceptions between us were resolved positively and amicably.

terms of the self-regulation of the profession. The onus is now on the profession to modernise self-regulation to maintain public confidence.' Yet we seemed to baulk when it came to decision time. It raised the spectre of the GMC of old – strong on the rhetoric, weak on execution.

The turning point had been the intervention of David Carter. Many people saw this also and were angry about his intervention. Others were jubilant; especially those opposed to revalidation. They saw the outcome as a great triumph. Undoubtedly and to some extent understandably, they felt that I had been justly rebuffed and repaid for leading affairs in this direction over the previous six months since the ending of the Bristol hearing.

Roddy MacSween and Richard Horton (the *Lancet* Editor) had both been in the gallery. Roddy had already spoken to some of the medical Royal College Presidents who were dismayed, particularly the surgeons. But overall the Colleges' immediate reaction was to press on, to take over the baton from the GMC if need be and to keep running with the revalidation agenda.

Roddy and I repaired for dinner. He was anxious about what would happen next and in particular whether I would lose heart and determination. But by this time I had recovered somewhat and was again feeling robust, seeing this as a setback, not a reverse. As we talked it through, we reminded ourselves of the incontrovertible fact that there were only two control mechanisms to ensure doctors' fitness to practise. One was through the doctors' contract (managerial), the other through registration (professional). Registration extended nationwide to every doctor, while contracts of employment affected only those in employment.

And then we had a really good conversation about pathology – Roddy was a liver histopathologist. He reminded me that there were only about 20 liver histopathologists in the country. So we talked about what it would actually mean in practice for histopathologists to be revalidated. What kind of evidence would be needed to demonstrate continuing competence? What was available in pathology from the various quality assurance arrangements the speciality had in place already on which pathologists could draw for evidence? He was very encouraging; there was a lot of good practice in place to build on.

People take up positions

There was a variety of reactions to the outcome. Overall the national press reactions were muted. Celia Hall in the *Daily Telegraph* thought that the GMC had 'pulled back from ordering regular competency checks on senior doctors'. Noting that the Council had voted that doctors should regularly demonstrate their fitness to practise, she added that it could not decide on the means of doing so. She noted that I, and other leaders of the medical profession, had been keen that the Council move quickly following the Bristol heart children's scandal. Sarah Bosely from the *Guardian* and Jeremy Lawrence (*Independent*) were both very perceptive and astute in their assessment of the politics, realising how much of a setback this was for the reformers.

The medical press was more outspoken. Richard Horton could not believe the result. When his leader in the *Lancet*[79] came out it spoke of those opposed to revalidation as 'yesterday's doctors' as an impediment to progress. He noted the extent to which the lay people on the Council had supported revalidation. The medical weeklies were at odds in their editorial comment. All were dismayed at the lack of a decision. *Doctor* magazine was strongly supportive of my line. *Hospital Doctor* – specialist oriented – was strongly critical of my line and basically said that I had blown it for the profession. So six of one and half a dozen of another in the same editorial stable!

And so, as that week came to a close, in my diary I questioned more than I had ever done before whether professional self-regulation as we know it was really viable. There could be no doubt about the need to incorporate medical technical expertise into the assessment of technical matters. But at the end of the day, it was the lay members and the appointed members of the Council who were most solidly supportive of the public interest, and it was amongst the elected majority that the doctor-centred attitudes were most on display. It was that protective focus amongst so many of the elected members, particularly amongst those prominent in the BMA, that I found most disconcerting.

My doubts were reinforced by the fact that in our Fitness to Practise committees we were still having an uphill struggle to bring about the fundamental reorientation necessary. Here, I noted in my diary, the real question was whether more efficient and effective processes, including more effective training of panel members, would of themselves bring about the necessary realignment towards public expectations. I reflected ruefully that variability of attitudes of elected members was still the potential Achilles' heel.

A week later and the repercussions could still be felt. I noted at the time that the lay members, in private conversation in particular, were dismayed by last week's affairs.

I saw Alan Milburn, now of course Secretary of State, on Wednesday 11 November. The meeting was primarily to talk about the 'Henry VIII' clause – the plan to put much of the regulatory arrangements for the health professions into secondary legislation. On this he was clearly as concerned about the regulation of the other health professions as he was about the GMC. Nevertheless, I introduced revalidation. He said he was surprised by the way the vote had gone the previous week and I agreed with him. I put it to him that we needed to know where he would stand on revalidation before we got to the February 1999 Conference which would consider the matter further. I reminded him that, in terms of securing the best protection for patients, the GMC's registration system was still the only mechanism for achieving a nationally consistent standard. And I reiterated our view of the importance of clinical governance at the local level and how decisions about the revalidation of registration should draw on doctors' performance data collected through appraisal. The two mechanisms – appraisal and revalidation – should be symbiotic, rather than stand alone.

I then had some reassuring meetings, pushing me back up the positive mood swing. I visited Trent that same day to talk at the NHS trusts chief executives' seminar. I had an hour and a quarter with the chief executives. This was on clinical governance and medical regulation. I set out the line and the difficulties and I noted their anxieties about their roles and in particular their responsibilities under the new clinical governance arrangements. Many of the chief executives were strong on the need for revalidation as a support to them. Without it, effective appraisal would be very difficult, if not impossible, to implement. The potential for wide variation within the hospitals and across trusts was too strong.

I felt similarly buoyed up when I met a group of the West Midlands Surgical Society and the East Midlands Surgical Society who were in conference at Burton-upon-Trent on Friday 13 November. There were about 80 surgeons there and they were all very anxious to hear about the Bristol implications for surgery, not least in the light of the RCS decision to revalidate. And they were confused and concerned about the ambiguity and the negative messages that had come from the GMC the week before. I was straight with them, but recognised their particular anxiety in surgery. I urged them not to step back from the revalidation issue. In the event there were good questions and some very positive expressions of goodwill afterwards. Several surgeons expressed disagreement, but all said they had appreciated the value of the personal contact and of having the chance to hear and question me at first hand in what was a very worrying time for them. This underlined for me the value of this sort of personal exposure. It was vital in learning what people felt on the ground, and also for talking it over with them personally.

The outside views continued to flow in. On Tuesday 17 November I spent the day at Cambridge visiting the medical school. That very day *The Times* published a leader, very critical of the medical profession, essentially questioning the ongoing viability of professional self-regulation. That was particularly important because of our perception that *The Times* closely mirrored government thinking.

In my diary I noted that the press coverage of the profession continued badly, with the analysis of the Ledward case and a meeting of patients who were calling for an independent inquiry into Ledward. We knew that government advisors were encouraging the press to look for other cases to publicise. This was not a good time for medicine.

Another go: the Internal Conference, 10 February 1999

Following the incomplete decisions in November 1998, we had to have a special conference – followed by a short formal Council – to adopt the principle of revalidation and extend that principle to all doctors through registration.[80] The paper discussed at the meeting introduced the idea of a staged model – local profiling, regular review, assessment and external quality assurance. The meeting included a number of outside speakers, for example Peter Hawker from the BMA consultants' committee, Sir William Wells (Chair of the Regional Health Authority Chairs), Nizam Mamode who was the Deputy Chairman of the Junior Doctors' Committee of the BMA and others.

There had been press comment, based on the papers pre-circulated with the Council, and the opponents seized upon this as an attempt to pre-empt the discussion. For example, Sarah Boseley had a very full report under the byline 'Doctors who fail new checks to be struck off' (Tuesday 2 February). She anticipated the size of the challenge in a further report in the *Guardian* on Wednesday 10 February under the byline 'Doctors to challenge competence checks plan'. She referred to 'a strong challenge . . . by a group of doctors opposed to the GMC's proposals to strike doctors off the Register if they fail to prove their fitness to practice'.

The Conference was to reveal a tetchiness amongst a minority who were opposed to revalidation from the outset. We had had very good forewarning of the possibly disruptive tactics that would be followed. Ed Borman, an anaesthetist member of the BMA CCSC as well as GMC Council Member, had his own paper and wished that to be admitted as an alternative. He got stuck into procedural argument within minutes of starting and the obstetrician, Wendy Savage, weighed in with him. But the meeting did not agree to admit papers that were not produced in time to be circulated beforehand and had therefore to be tabled on the day.

Ed Borman, who strongly supported the principles of clinical governance, but not of the linkage with registration, continued to question the need: 'Could someone please explain how revalidation . . . will be derived and what that is going to add, without having problems of legal challenge?' He reflected a genuine concern that had been raised by others outside the GMC who were questioning the need for revalidation.

Nevertheless, supporters of revalidation had made their own plans and the general direction of the debate was positive. A key factor in the process was to have small-group discussions before holding the general discussion. This had given more people more time to work their thoughts through. Anthony Grabham voiced his concerns about doctors who would not co-operate. We clarified the point that no doctor would lose their registration without going through the formal performance procedures unless they refused to give any evidence in the first place. In these circumstances the doctor could automatically lose their registration as a doctor, as they already could by not maintaining an up-to-date address.

Roddy MacSween reaffirmed the Academy's acceptance of the principle of revalidation and their desire to see it dovetailed into local processes. An early speaker was Peter Hawker from whom I had expected opposition. He spoke of the major contributions his committee had been making to develop national systems to deal with poorly performing doctors, especially in the past year when looking at appraisal and professional development. He referred to the fact that the debate on revalidation had caused an enormous amount of concern and that one could not pretend otherwise. The initial anxiety had reflected the belief that revalidation would mean an examination, which might lead to loss of the right to practise. That, he was now quite clear, was not on the agenda. He referred also to a lot of anxiety about the detail – how it would all actually work.

But he was unequivocal in his own position on that occasion:

> I will now clearly state – and I will take the responsibility and flack which will occur at the committee meeting which is due in a few weeks' time – that as Chairman of my committee, representing my colleagues, I give my personal and my committee's full support to the Steering Group's proposal. I further associate myself very firmly with the letter that Dr Bogle wrote to you with some, I believe, helpful comments.

Liam Donaldson (CMO, England) was equally positive. He said:

> Both myself and the Department of Health as a whole would like very warmly to welcome these proposals. They have our full support. We see no devil in the detail. We see a lot of hard work to get the implementation right.

He added that his personal support for revalidation came from having been involved in the original conceptualisation of clinical governance:

. . . recognising that it was only a concept and that there were important parts of it that needed to be filled in. One of the clear deficits was to introduce a strong element of professional accountability, which was missing. So I see this [revalidation] as an important piece of the overall framework of quality in the NHS which needs to be, and must be, put in place.

He had two comments on implementation, namely, the strong interdependence between professional self-regulation – of which this was an important part – and clinical governance and the statutory duty of quality within the NHS. His second comment referred to the potential for contributing not just to quality assurance but also to quality improvement. He saw a dynamic feature there:

Going hand in hand, I think that clinical governance, revalidation and professional self-regulation as a whole are two major engines that can drive change in quality improvement in the NHS – and this is an opportunity that we cannot miss.

Gill Markham had revised her position. She now felt reassured about the need for the link with registration and believed 'that if we are doing this for public reassurance we need to involve all doctors from day one'. That of course was entirely consistent with the Council's belief that *Good Medical Practice* applied to all doctors.

And so she triggered the important transition that was made from a form of revalidation which was effectively re-certification, to the revalidation of the basic Register itself – re-licensure. Finlay Scott was certainly aware of the practical consequences of this: the huge amount of work entailed; the GMC's consequential dependence on others putting systems in place; and the opportunity there would have been for a phased introduction by starting with the two big groups originally envisaged – specialists and general practitioners. Practically he was right, but I was content with this step, for re-licensure had always seemed to me the logical conclusion if one was talking about the basic integrity of the Register, as I had said in my letter to the GMC in 1988 (*see* Chapter 6).

Dr Surendra Kumar, Chair of the Overseas Doctors' Association, welcomed revalidation. Referring to the evidence required, he favoured the use of patient satisfaction surveys as a means of enhancing public confidence, but he was anxious about the human resources needed to make it all work.

Barbara Meredith was a guest from the National Consumer Council. She spoke about the need to make the public better aware of what was going on, to make the public better informed. She noted that a lot of the professional reaction to the revalidation proposal had been based on fear – 'you will be struck off if you do not do it' – rather than the proactive aspect of systemising and giving some coherence to things like clinical audit and continuing professional development. She mentioned the importance of extending the jurisdiction to doctors in the private sector – which of course registration does – and the importance of involving lay and patient views when considering outcomes and setting standards for clinical audit.

Sir William Wells wanted to refute the point made to him on several occasions, that revalidation could be separated from clinical governance and vice versa. In his view and that of his colleagues in NHS management, they were an integral part of each other. He went on to say that:

> We [the Regional Chairs] have told the Secretary of State, given that we have the responsibility for delivering clinical governance through the boards of all the various health establishments which are responsible, that it will be very difficult to deliver the full element of clinical governance without having revalidation. I believe, one step further, that revalidation has to have teeth and therefore has to be linked to registration. If you do not do that, it will not be seen by the public as being anything other than just a palliative . . . . If we really believe in clinical governance – and I think there is a very strong belief in clinical governance – then we have no other option but to introduce revalidation linked to registration. If we do not, then the consequences are quite clear: something else will have to be put in its place.

Wendy Savage supported Gill Markham's view that revalidation should apply to all doctors from the beginning but added that it should only be implemented if and when the resources needed had been identified. She also objected to the use of the word 'revalidation', which 'crept into the November Council without any definition, which now has a definition'.* She would have preferred the word 'accreditation'.

John Chisholm spoke strongly for the BMA's General Practitioners' Committee and the RCGP both of which favoured a process of re-accreditation or re-certification. He felt that 'to rely on the process of clinical governance would be insufficient, because essentially that is a process that only applies within the NHS, and the GMC has the duty to protect the public in respect of all doctors on the Medical Register'. He referred to the multiplicity of professional and other bodies that would be involved in the process, and of course the fear of general practitioners about time and resources.

Joyce Struthers (Association of Community Health Councils) acknowledged the value of the essentially local process of evidence collection

---

* I had used the word 'revalidation' before on occasions, as an umbrella word covering 're-certification' and 're-licence'. I did not know until someone drew my attention to it, that the word did not exist in the English language. It does now!

and appraisal, but she counselled against rubber-stamping by the GMC. She wanted to be assured that this would not be the case.

Bob Nicholls (lay member) spoke warmly about the positive reception from outside guests. He was a powerful and very public supporter of self-regulation. But as a former NHS manager, he countered Liam Donaldson's statements by cautioning against too close a fusion between the professional and managerial processes: 'If you want self-regulation, the profession has to demonstrate that it is doing it, and that its standards are national and across the whole piece.'

Linda Patterson (GMC member and an NHS Trust Medical Director) was strongly in favour of the proposals and asserted that it would assist her in her work, particularly in dealing with poorly performing doctors: 'It is really important that we engage trusts, health authorities and regional offices with what we're about; that we match up those processes. Otherwise there could be parallel systems starting up which could produce a lot of tension.'*

Jim Johnson (Joint Consultants' Committee; JCC) said that he was delighted with the huge level of support for the principles discussed that day:

> After the November meeting, the public perceptions were that the GMC had wobbled . . . . When anyone explained precisely why the resolutions that were passed had been passed, it made eminent good sense; but, as you all know, that was not how it was reported in the press nor was it how it was seen elsewhere, not least in Parliament.

Noting that much important detail would have to be sorted out, he nevertheless said that, for the outside world, the big picture that must go out today was that the GMC overwhelmingly supported the principles of the paper.

Jenny Simpson from the British Association of Medical Managers explained that medical directors and clinical directors, the people responsible for making the appraisal of doctors' work, thought that they could not do the job without revalidation.

For me, GMC member David Hatch put the real positive purpose of revalidation very simply. He said:

> I was appointed a consultant anaesthetist at Great Ormond Street [The Hospital for Sick Children] in 1969. In that 30 years nobody has given me an opportunity to demonstrate that I am fit to practise and up to date. I would welcome the opportunity to try to show that to the parents of the children I anaesthetise and the children themselves in

---

* Of course this perception was to develop later with the trial run of the first revalidation folders.

some cases. I would hope that the [Medical] Register, available 24 hours a day, seven days a week, would be the instrument for doing that. I hope that people will look up the Register, and the fact that I am on it will indicate that I am safe to anaesthetise their children.

I can imagine that the parents of the Bristol children would say 'Amen' to that.

At the Council meeting the same day[81] the formal resolutions were passed. The motion linking revalidation to registration was carried (62 votes for, 5 against, 14 abstentions). The decision to extend revalidation to include all registered doctors and the use of the Fitness to Practise procedures as the backstop in cases of serious dysfunction were also carried, both with no votes against and four abstentions.

So the stage was set for the development of the working model of revalidation on which the GMC would consult in due course. And the decision was decisive. Whew!

12

The Shipman impact

The decision of the February Conference was important for several reasons. About three-quarters of the Council had voted in favour of the revalidation proposals with only a very small core – mainly of BMA Council members – voting against. This demonstrated the size of the majority in the GMC in favour of this basic reform. I saw revalidation as the touchstone because it went to the heart of the change in culture that every doctor had to make.

This was a difficult time for doctors. Still reeling from the public and press reactions to the profession following Bristol and Ledward, in short order, doctors were confused. I was travelling a lot and met many. Hospital doctors I spoke to were feeling particularly bruised because of the perceived devaluing of their professionalism and the perception that the government was gunning for them. Increased accountability, especially when put alongside increased workload, was a real problem for them.

There was growing unease at the signs that the GMC was becoming more assertively protective of patients and less likely therefore to come down on the side of the doctor against whom a complaint had been made. I used to hear doctors say that the GMC is not 'representing us' any more. Perception is all. In fact in this period of rapidly increasing numbers of cases – mainly clinical – the proportion of doctors who were erased actually began to fall. But the absolute numbers increased and these were the cases that attracted attention in the press, giving the impression of a much harder line. Add to this revalidation and one can fully understand.

The national press, partly of its own volition and partly stimulated by the agencies of government,* continued to focus on the GMC as an ineffective regulator. That was not difficult to do, for in addition to Bristol

---

* Our private intelligence was sure of their spin.

and Ledward, harrowing stories of women damaged after treatment by another gynaecologist, Richard Neale, were being widely publicised. Indeed they gave evidence before the House of Commons Select Committee on Health in June, and there was a BBC *Panorama* programme on Neale on 1 March which made deeply disturbing viewing (*see* Chapter 14). In September Harold Shipman, a family doctor in Hyde, Greater Manchester, was charged with the murder of an elderly patient, Mrs Kathleen Grundy. More awful revelations about his practice soon followed. Meanwhile, the profession – especially in the hospital service – was beginning to protest with increasing vociferousness that it was being victimised and asked to cope with the effects of new regulation and clinical governance at a time when the clinical workload had never been higher.

In the summer of 1999, there was an ITV *Cook Report* on the restorations of doctors to the Medical Register after being found guilty of SPM. It described gruesome cases, reinforcing the impressions of the 1998 *Dispatches* programme on the GMC's apparently erratic approach to erasure from the Register, and its willingness to re-register some doctors who subsequently erred again. Actually figures showed that the majority of doctors struck off never practised again. But the law enabled a doctor who had been struck off to apply again for restoration to the Medical Register after only 10 months. In the programme, cases were produced where doctors who had committed serious misconduct were restored to the register quite quickly – within two or three years. In the minds of the public and government, a tighter policy on restorations to the Register therefore became a fundamental issue in seeking safer professional regulation. The fact that the GMC had been pressing for a change in the law and could do little about the situation without government making such a change was not highlighted. The profession was not fully persuaded of the GMC line. Indeed the pressure for a tighter GMC policy on erasures and restorations revealed real difficulties – such is the issue of rehabilitation versus punishment – which were fully explored in the subsequent Council debates. It illustrated the tension between public and professional expectations, and genuine differences of opinion about the purpose of erasure – is it simply to protect the public? Is it to send a message about unacceptable behaviour? Does it include an element of punishment?

Against all this it is important to remember the two powerful, ongoing, positive threads. First, the determination of government, the majority of the GMC and most in the medical profession to reform and modernise the GMC. Second, the determination of the GMC itself to create the framework for the needed change in the culture of medicine, a culture exemplified in *Good Medical Practice*, clinical governance and revalidation.

The challenge to my presidency

One indication of the strength of opposition of what one might call the anti-reform group within the BMA was the challenge to my presidency in May 1999. Presidents are elected by the Council. A presidential term may be anything up to but not exceeding seven years. Council members are elected on a quinquennial basis. Any President who seeks to serve more than four or so years must therefore put themselves forward for re-election. There was no precedent for a mid-term challenge. But these were unprecedented times.

I first learnt about the possibility that Sandy Macara was considering standing from Ian Bogle when I met him for dinner on 20 January 1999 – six months after Bristol. Macara, a local colleague and friend of James Wisheart and at that time deeply opposed to revalidation, had been very critical of the GMC's involvement in the Bristol case. Now, I was told, he was thinking about standing for President of the GMC because of his unhappiness with the direction in which I was leading the Council.

But in the ensuing months his alleged challenge disappeared for reasons I have never understood, to give way to another candidate, Wendy Savage. In her election address, she said she had decided to stand because of her 'concerns about the manner and direction in which Sir Donald is leading us', concerns which she said were shared privately by others. Her key objections were to my actions in relation to Bristol and the 'haste with which revalidation was pushed through without adequate consultation'. She wanted change to continue but the profession must be fully involved and it must be based on good evidence of what is effective. Costs must be calculated and concrete plans made for raising the necessary money to develop sound, fair and just procedures. Caring for doctors and patients should be the way forward.

I was not surprised by Wendy's challenge. As I understood it the real issue was revalidation. She represented a perfectly legitimate alternative view in the profession, which wanted to go more slowly. In my own address I simply asked for support for the continuation of the reform programme. I won the election with a comfortable majority (56 to 26 with six abstentions*). I interpreted the result as a positive endorsement of the current reform policies. A bigger margin of success might have suggested that I was not being radical enough!

But, nevertheless, it was an indication of how things could change as the reality of revalidation and its significance for doctors really started to sink home. And there were lessons to be learned, particularly about the need for good communication on a subject as controversial as the accountability of doctors.

* It is a puzzle to me that people can abstain in these clear issues.

Parallel developments

In spite of this, during that summer and autumn of 1999 we maintained the pressures on internal development work. The overhaul of the Fitness to Practise procedures continued. Screening was being restructured and new screening guidance developed. Nevertheless the delays in handling complaints and getting cases heard was getting worse because of the huge increase in the numbers and complexity, particularly of those alleging poor clinical care. Preparations were being made to have the law changed on erasures and restorations. Much to everyone's relief the first performance cases were standing up well to legal scrutiny. The GMC and the other regulating bodies had campaigned successfully, with considerable parliamentary support, to secure the benefits but limit the adverse effects of what was called 'the Henry VIII' clause being brought before Parliament by the government (*see* Chapter 7). The GMC, the medical profession and the other professional regulators all supported the government's idea that much quicker change could be achieved using such enabling legislation. But we were opposed to the idea that changes to the fundamental nature and purpose of the regulators could be made without first having full parliamentary scrutiny and debate. We did not challenge the right of Parliament to make such changes if it chose to, only that such changes should first be properly tested and fully understood.

For the GMC it was also a time of enhancing relationships with the medical Royal Colleges. On 20 July 1999 we had the first joint meeting between the Academy of Medical Royal Colleges and the GMC, an initiative for which Roddy MacSween and myself were responsible. He and I believed that a far closer working relationship between the GMC and the Colleges was essential. We believed they, the Colleges, had a vital role in determining the professional standards for their specialities, and in future the clinical evidence that would be needed to demonstrate compliance with such standards for appraisal and revalidation.

Meanwhile, the Colleges were making progress with the task of producing their own interpretation of *Good Medical Practice*. They had been asked to produce versions that reflected the specific needs and standards of their own speciality, to ensure it was as appropriate and meaningful as possible for all aspects of medicine. Led by Professor David Hatch the anaesthetists were first over the line. The RCGP and the General Practitioners' Committee of the BMA went furthest because they described excellent and unacceptable practice.

Poorly performing doctors

The temperature was raised by the publication in September 1999 of a consultation paper, *Supporting Doctors, Protecting Patients,*[65] by the government on poorly performing doctors. This paper, prepared by Liam Donaldson, proposed that the NHS establish a new National Clinical Assessment Authority (NCAA) in England specifically for the purpose of assessing the competence of poorly performing doctors at their place of work. This caused huge anxiety amongst doctors in England, an anxiety shared in Scotland, Wales and Northern Ireland also. Over the ensuing months there was considerable opposition focused around what would become known as 'boot camps', centres to which allegedly poorly performing doctors would be referred. These centres would be local, and carry out an assessment of the doctor at their place of work, with referral onwards to the GMC in those cases where a doctor's registration would be questioned. There were those who saw this as a direct threat to the GMC's own performance procedures, just becoming established. The matter was aggravated by the Secretary of State, Alan Milburn, who seemed to regard these assessments as the definitive answer to anything to do with the dysfunctional doctor. In the event the NCAA took a constructive view and did not follow the 'boot camp' route.

It was six months before the argument over this gradually subsided. The GMC, in its response to the consultation paper, proposed that it might be more practical and effective to carry out assessments in much strengthened postgraduate deaneries. But the Department apparently had only limited confidence in deaneries and so this proposal was quietly sidelined.

It was really tricky to align all the new procedures. Some were going to be operated professionally, others managerially. They needed to interlock in a complementary and facilitative fashion, to provide a seamless way of identifying and acting promptly and effectively on dysfunctional doctors. The GMC tried to help this process by making its own assessment methodologies for poorly performing doctors available to the NCAA and in providing training facilities for NCAA assessors.

There is no doubt that some in government believed that the new managerial systems would replace the professional machinery for assessment just being established. But saner heads prevailed as the different but complementary functions of accountability through employment and accountability through registration became more readily understood (*see also* Chapter 15).

Liam and I differed only over this particular piece of the difficult interface between the managerial and professional systems. But the outcome was satisfactory. Neither of us ever wavered from our common central purpose – to see effective clinical governance established in clinical teams, supported by effective professional regulation within a comprehensive system for improving and assuring quality in healthcare.

Establishing new relationships

As the government established its new agencies the GMC started to develop new working relationships with the new bodies. On 7 September 1999 I had an excellent meeting with Deirdre Hine, formerly CMO Wales, and Peter Homa, a former Chief Executive of an NHS trust. They had been appointed Chairman and Chief Executive respectively of the new Commission for Health Improvement (CHI). The government originally had in mind a lay person for the Chair but in the event Deirdre was clearly the strongest candidate.

Both she and Peter had a clear vision for the new Commission. They believed that it should be constructive and positive in its broad approach, seeking to help bring about quality improvement in individual trusts and health authorities. Behind the scenes there had been a fair old tussle involving ministers and No. 10 about two opposing philosophies. There were those who wanted a new 'OFSTED' for the NHS. These were the hawkish controllers, the 'namers and shamers'. And there were the 'quality-improvers' like Deirdre and Peter. For the moment the quality, improving philosophy won. But that underlying tension was never far from the surface and remains so.

Subsequently informal working relationships were established between the GMC and CHI following that meeting, and excellent practical relationships evolved at staff level very quickly. These culminated in a formal memorandum of understanding. CHI had the job of looking at institutional quality, including the institutional arrangements for regulating doctors at their place of work. The GMC had the professional job of being sure about the competence and integrity of individual doctors who were registered with it. In practical terms the new working relationship meant that where the CHI became involved in an investigation in which it appeared that matters to do with the professionalism of an individual doctor were at issue, the GMC would become involved. Conversely there were situations where the GMC, in the course of investigating a complaint, would come across matters to do with institutional governance and management which appeared to need further enquiry. These it would refer informally to the Commission.

So, through this collaboration at the regulator level, really new and effective partnerships began to be formed. Co-ordinated regulation was beginning to take shape on the ground, where it mattered most.

Shipman: serial killer

Harold Shipman, a trusted popular general practitioner, qualified in 1970 and entered partnership in general practice in 1974. In 1992 he set up in single-handed practice in Hyde. In that small community he was respected by many, and loved by some of his patients. Between 1995 and 1998 he murdered 15 patients, none of them with serious terminal illness. All were women, all were killed by lethal doses of diamorphine administered in the patients' own homes or his surgery. Sometimes relations or surgery staff were close by, even in the next room.

To cover his tracks, clinical records and death certificates were falsified. Detection took some time because he was so trusted, and indeed his activities only came to light when he falsified the will of one of the patients he had killed. The police wrote to the GMC in 1998 to alert us that Shipman was being investigated for murder, and on 1 October the GMC was informed that he had been charged with murder on 7 September. The GMC was criticised at the time for not suspending him during his trial. However the GMC could not, by law, use its emergency powers of suspension once a doctor was charged with a criminal offence, until a final resolution was achieved.

Shipman was convicted of murder at Preston on 31 January 2000. Immediately the GMC started emergency proceedings and on Friday 11 February he was formally struck off the Medical Register.

He had a previous history with the GMC. In 1976 he was convicted of dishonestly obtaining drugs and forging NHS prescriptions. Both the courts and the GMC dealt with him leniently, regarding him as in need of treatment rather than punishment. Psychiatrists who saw him then for the GMC believed that he had overcome what they regarded as a personal drug problem. He was issued with a warning by the GMC.

Subsequently in 2001 the DoH published a review of Harold Shipman's clinical practice between 1974 and 1998. In July 2002, the public inquiry published its first report.[82] It concluded that 215 patients were unlawfully killed and that a 'real suspicion' remained over 45 others.

Shipman's was the ultimate and most shocking betrayal of trust. There were clearly lessons to be learned about death and cremation certificates, the scrutiny of single-handed practice, the integrity of medical records, the monitoring of death rates and the control of unused controlled drugs. The government responded to the GMC's request to close the loophole in the law preventing the GMC from suspending a doctor on a criminal charge.

I said at the time that I believed that the new arrangements for the regular scrutiny of a doctor's practice – appraisal and revalidation – could help prevent what has to be a quite exceptional type of crime. But no system could ever be 100% safe. As Cecil Clothier had said in his report on the nurse, Beverly Allitt, 'a determined and secret criminal may defeat the best regulated organisation in the pursuit of his or her purpose'. Shipman was a serial killer who systematically abused the trust placed in him, and the opportunities his position and training as a doctor provided.

Alan Milburn made a statement to the House immediately after Shipman's conviction. His statement had a strong steer for the GMC on the need for it to review its procedures and direction, and in particular that it had to be unequivocal about being there primarily to protect patients. I thought that the statement would be helpful in terms of reinforcing the need for reform amongst the sections of the medical profession which were still sceptical.

The following day, Thursday 3 February, I had a meeting with Alan Milburn at Richmond House. This had been pre-arranged for some time and regularly postponed no doubt to await the end of the Shipman trial. I had Finlay Scott with me and Alan Milburn had Simon Stevens, his political advisor, and one of his officials.

It was a sparky conversation, in which he seemed to be saying that the GMC was responsible for most of the ills of the system. I reminded him firmly of the huge failures that there had been in NHS management at Bristol, in the case of Rodney Ledward and, as was already clear, in Shipman too. It was simply not acceptable or helpful to dump it all on the profession and its regulator. I tried unsuccessfully to bring him back to the substance of the modernising agenda but he did not seem to be listening. It was an experience of Alan Milburn being unreasonable.

And so it ended, but not before we had restored a more positive attitude to what needed to be done. I told him as we were leaving that what we really required was a new Medical Act, to complete the reforms already underway, particularly in Fitness to Practise. We both knew there needed to be a new, smaller GMC. I told him that I would be asking the GMC to press on with these reforms with the utmost sense of urgency. I was opposed to any form of independent inquiry such as the nurses had had (it was not suggested), and which had led to the setting up of the new Nursing and Midwifery Council. I believed that the best result in the long run would be achieved if the GMC and its principal stakeholders worked out the way forward themselves, rather than have solutions imposed from outside. He asked me how long it would take and when my presidency was due to end. I said that I would want to have the main framework agreed with the stakeholders – the profession, the patients' organisations, the employers and the government – before I left office in about two years' time. As we left Richmond House Finlay said to me, 'I could see his mind working out exactly how long you had left to get these changes through.'

Finlay and I left that meeting determined in our own minds that we would indeed redouble our efforts in the GMC to get professional regulation right for patients by cracking the outstanding and biggest defects in our system. But I was under no illusion, as I noted in my diary at the time. I felt at that time that Alan Milburn's approach was all part of a wider political game. This involved the government's broader thinking about professional regulation, about getting more control over general practice, about cutting the over-mighty doctors down to size and shifting the spotlight away from the NHS's role in the Shipman affair. At the same time this would divert attention from the heat the government was already feeling from the public and the profession over NHS resources. We were all getting wise to the spin!

I could understand some of the pressures on government. In that same winter, there was a winter bed crisis in the NHS. On 12 January, Robert Winston had published an outburst in the *New Statesman*, criticising the government heavily for the under-resourcing of the NHS. Then on 16 January, Tony Blair gave an interview on the *Frost Programme* in which he announced suddenly huge increases in investment for the NHS. I cannot remember a previous occasion when such a huge policy change in direction was announced on a chat show on a Sunday morning. I saw in that action a hint of panic, as did many others. In the budget later in the spring the full dimension of the £2 billion per year was then re-announced in more measured tones by the Chancellor.

One further thought on that meeting with Milburn. Despite his anger that day, I believed that he was fully behind my plans for GMC reform, insofar as these linked in with his own. The big question mark was over the GMC itself.* Was it sufficiently cohesive and progressive to bring about the kind of changes that were needed against what were perceived to be very strong forces of resistance within the profession and in the GMC itself?

The GMC Conference, 8 February 2000

It was indeed fortunate that the GMC was having a special two-day conference so shortly after the upheaval caused by the Shipman verdict. This was a new Council and I knew that members were particularly keen to have the opportunity of a 'blue skies' session in which they could contemplate the future. And there were further parts of the modernisation of Fitness to Practise which had to be dealt with, particularly the business of getting the law changed, so that people could be brought in from outside to help service Fitness to Practise committees.

But in view of the wider political situation I asked the Council to put aside the agenda so that we could discuss the immediate issues. I

---

* I learnt much later that in both Richmond House and 10 Downing St, regular estimates were made by advisors as to likely voting intentions of members of the GMC on the reform programme, and therefore the likelihood of the programme being carried through successfully.

reported on the outcome of my discussions with Alan Milburn and about the absolute necessity of pressing on at the highest possible speed with our programme of reform. To my surprise some thought that we should not be deflected from our agenda by outside political events. That provoked 20 minutes of argument while the pros and cons of this were discussed. I was much relieved when Ruth Evans stood up and said that she could hardly believe what she was hearing. This was exactly the dysfunctional, out-of-touch GMC that the public were complaining about. 'Listen to the President and support what he is saying', she urged.

And so we moved into a very wide-ranging discussion – ragged in many places – in which almost everybody had their say during the course of the day. It was all about future direction. It was good to hear from new members, many of whom seemed quite clear that further change was needed and that we should get on with it. There was general support for the idea that we should be more radical in our thinking on Fitness to Practise. We established a working group to take that forward. There was more mixed support for the proposal that we should have a working group on the governance and structure of the GMC which government was insisting on. The conservatives on the Council were particularly resistant to this, anxious not to be knee-jerked by either the government or the press into what they thought could be an unnecessary reaction.

On the second day I held a press conference at lunchtime. By the end of that morning I had got a clear sense of direction from the Council, particularly for increasing the proportion of lay members on the GMC and of establishing the two policy reform groups. This gave me the authority I needed to be really positive at the press conference itself. There was a large turnout. There were a lot of searching questions, particularly about whether this was a GMC reaction to the government statement, and whether the GMC was really changing its outlook and culture. As a result of robust and clear briefing, there was a generally good response and good feedback from the press the following day.

Meanwhile, more on restorations

As I told Mr Milburn at our heated meeting in February, the GMC had written to the Minister seeking legislative change to the unacceptable position under the current Medical Act, whereby a doctor who was struck off the Register was entitled by law to apply for restoration within 10 months.* The GMC had had several thoughtful, high-quality

* The Committee hearing the application for restoration would not necessarily be that which made the original decision, and if the doctor brought evidence of development and change it was often difficult to refuse, so restorations were a problem.

discussions on this and had pressed the DoH for some years to change the legislation to require a doctor to wait for three years before being allowed to make any application for restoration.

Later in February a letter from Alan Milburn arrived giving notice that he would make a five-year minimum for restorations. The Council had debated the appropriate length of time – five years or three – and concluded that three would be more likely to give the best practical result. It would avoid the pressure that would otherwise arise in panels considering erasure actually to hold back if they thought that the doctor would never be able to return.* The rehabilitation element of any sanction would be harmed and potentially useful members of a scarce profession would be lost.

Of course technically there was an inherent inconsistency in our policy. If a return to the Register should be exceptional – a doctor who was erased should have no expectation of return – then the length of time was really immaterial. Alan Milburn was right when he alluded to that inconsistency when he referred in the letter to the legislation 'you say you need'. His view was that a determined profession would not need the law to be changed – it had all the powers it needed if it chose to use them. I agreed with his view. My own personal belief was that public trust in the system would be most likely to be sustained if GMC committees looking at applications for restoration to the Register took a relatively hard line on those whom an earlier panel had judged to be unfit to be in the medical profession. But if, as with prison sentences, there was a belief that people could change, then it was important to get the balance right between protection and the marking of misconduct on the one hand, and rehabilitation and reform on the other. It was another good example of the unresolved tension in the culture between those who believed in restitution if possible – almost in spite of the nature of the original misconduct – and those like myself who believed that a doctor who had 'blown it' sufficient to be thrown out of the profession should have no expectation of return.

We would come back to Alan Milburn's point time and again as things unfolded. We became far more aware that the GMC, if it had a different attitude, had in fact already got powers to take a much tougher line on safety measures if it chose to do so. The same could be said incidentally of NHS authorities, which I had long believed could have done more about poor practice if they had chosen to do so. It came down once again to will. The GMC needed the explicit powers, of course, to make sure that its members acted consistently and as firmly as desirable. We had the same kind of argument about defining serious professional misconduct. Endless

* After five years out of clinical practice, a doctor would be virtually obliged to return to at least pre-registration year training to prove themselves competent and fit to practise.

hours have been spent on this over the years. Should misconduct be qualified by the word 'serious'? What does serious actually mean? But of course the GMC actually has the power to make it mean what it wants to make it mean. That was what Alan Milburn was getting at and he was quite right. So we needed a new kind of thinking. Decide what is the right thing to do. Make sure the law enables you to do it. If it does not, change it. But abandon the traditional reason for not acting by hiding behind poor law, and blaming lack of action when challenged on that law. More cultural change!

13

A profession divided

The year 2000 turned out to be the GMC's *annus horribilis*. Or, looking at it more positively, the year when the medical profession finally confronted the realities of cultural change, and, for the majority, came to terms with these, albeit somewhat reluctantly. The Shipman murders were used by the government to push for wider change in general practice. But there was deep anger in the profession with the implication that Shipman's murderous character was somehow linked to his being a doctor.

Fuses shortened in the summer with the arrival of two further case drivers for change – the GMC hearing of Richard Neale and the outcome of the independent inquiry on Ledward.[77] The balloon went up. Between June 2000 and the summer of 2001 things were critical for the GMC and the profession. It is the story of that crisis that I turn to next. As the saga unfolds, it is worthwhile keeping in mind the following points. Of the three major reforms now brought forward, the most ambitious was revalidation for reasons that will become clear. Although there were anxieties across the profession, general practice and the specialist Royal Colleges were basically in support. The focus of opposition was in the BMA's Consultants and Specialists Committee and angst amongst some of the hospital juniors.

The second issue was the future constitution and governance of the GMC, the first priority of the government. Here opinions were much more divided across all sectors of the profession. The third was the reform of the Fitness to Practise procedures, at least as important but less contentious because the profession, the GMC, patient organisations and government were all much closer together on what needed to be done. But, behind all this were much deeper issues about professional power and control, particularly over lay involvement in future regulatory processes in the GMC and elsewhere, issues that have run throughout this story so far. In a sense that is where the real cultural change was happening.

BMA resistance emerges

At the end of February 2000 my wife and I left for a conference on medical regulation in Cape Town, to be followed by our annual holiday. A BMA Council meeting was imminent. I left knowing that discontent was rising within the BMA consultants' committee about revalidation and that there were wider justified concerns about the continued delays in getting Fitness to Practise cases heard. These delays were the consequence partly of the antiquated procedures that were still being changed and partly the relentlessly rising number of complaints about doctors to the GMC. Some BMA Council members were also GMC Council members. Ironically, it was some of these who were so critical of the GMC yet themselves tardy in supporting the kind of changes the GMC needed to make to overcome the shortage of members to serve on Fitness to Practise committees and to streamline processes, to achieve an effective reduction of the backlog.

I rang Ian Bogle, the BMA Chairman, from Cape Town on Wednesday 1 March to find out how the BMA Council had gone. He was full of doom and gloom and said that it had gone badly for the GMC. The debate had focused around a critical motion put by Sam Everington, a general practitioner. This had opened the floodgates for a general attack on the GMC and, from about four people, on myself. As I understood it, the general thrust of the criticisms was about the delay in getting cases heard and about some of the decisions of the PCC which appeared to go against doctors. The general description by those attacking was of a GMC that was inefficient and not sufficiently protective of doctors' legitimate interests. The result was an instruction from the BMA Council to the BMA's GMC subcommittee to come up with a plan for reform before the next BMA Council meeting in May. Ian reminded me that 'many of your enemies are in the GMC itself'. However, as we talked it through it became clear that the general practitioners on the BMA Council – with the exception of Sam Everington – had been stronger in support than the specialists. Despite Ian's assurances that revalidation was not a factor, I thought that it nevertheless probably underlay a lot of the specialist objections.

I spoke subsequently on the telephone to several BMA Council members who were equally gloomy about the meeting, describing the tide of abuse about the GMC as just about the worst possible thing the BMA could have condoned at the moment of trying to advance serious reform. Denis Pereira Gray (Academy) said that the critical messages were not consistent. Some members wanted an end to self-regulation, others wanted a different model, and yet others were just anxious about the profession being attacked by the government over Shipman.

I learnt that at the BMA press conference that morning Ian Bogle had himself been very critical of the GMC and of my own leadership, noting that the GMC was 'strong on vision' but that the plans for delivery were vague and that he did not fully understand them. He told the press that he had spoken to me 'in no uncertain terms' about this situation. When I challenged him on this reportage later I sensed discomfort. He said that he had merely been reporting how others at the meeting had felt.

Subsequent to the BMA Council, there was a meeting of the Joint Consultants' Committee in which there were, I understand, attacks on the GMC and on myself, led by Sandy Macara and Ed Borman, the same people – particularly about my leadership.

Sally and I had the weekend in Cape Town and then reluctantly cut our holiday to return to London. I attended a meeting of the government's Better Regulation Task Force on Thursday 9 March when I had another insight into consultant thinking. Jim Johnson, Chairman of the Joint Consultants' Committee, was there. He told this very mixed meeting how doctors were feeling harassed, how important self-regulation was to doctors, but that they feared the GMC. This reflected his and his colleagues' line at other meetings, particularly in the revalidation meetings at the GMC. Clearly the idea of a new order of accountability to the profession's regulator was a harder pill for some specialists to swallow than it was for GPs. However it was also clear that the specialists themselves were becoming more divided, particularly over the revalidation issue. The medical Royal Colleges were sticking to their line of supporting the GMC on revalidation.

On 15 March the BMA asked for a meeting which was held at the BMA's headquarters in Tavistock Square. Peter Hawker, the consultants' Chairman, started by saying that the profession intended to keep self-regulation but not necessarily through the GMC. Then he complained – clearly a spillover from the recent BMA Council meeting – about the slowness of the GMC and the loss of confidence in it by the profession. Derek Machin, his Vice Chairman, was particularly unpleasant and personally insulting. His complaint was that we were not doing sufficient to protect doctors from the public and that in particular I danced too easily to the government's tune.

Although the meeting was ostensibly about revalidation we hardly touched on it, for it mainly covered these wider issues. But when we returned to it, the subject was clearly the real cause of anxiety and anger. The personal attacks on me – as with most personal attacks I find – felt like substitutes for logical and rational arguments about genuine disagreements about policy. But we agreed that further talks would be helpful.

On Wednesday 22 March I met Sheila McKechnie, the Director of the Consumers' Association, Clara McKay and Sally Williams who were the senior policy researchers at the Association. The Consumers' Association was critical of the GMC's past performance and its current attitudes to complainants. But they were critical in a constructive way, for they supported the direction of travel of the reforms. Clara and Sally very much favoured the idea of co-regulation rather than professionally led regulation. Sheila wanted to be sure that lay members of the GMC would be appointed by a more independent body than the DoH. Both liked the idea of the GMC as a point of partnership between the medical profession and the public. What they were looking for and what the BMA were looking for were in some important respects completely at odds as things currently stood.

On Thursday 23 March there was a further discussion at the BMA, mainly on revalidation. It was a much more measured and paced meeting, and one sensed that perhaps some of the fire had died down. Isabel Nisbet, at that time our new Director of Fitness to Practise, had gone there expecting there to be blood on the floor!

Meanwhile, the discussions with the general practitioners over revalidation were still going well. The GPC of the BMA was cautious but nevertheless clear about direction. Its main concerns were about resources, including the time to do assessment and appraisal properly. The RCGP that was leading on revalidation development in general practice was doing a tremendous job, developing the general practice version of *Good Medical Practice* and objective approaches to assessment and professional development – Accredited Professional Development (APD). They and their GPC colleagues had formed a very effective partnership, for which much credit goes to the two Chairmen, Mike Pringle (RCGP) and John Chisholm (GPC). I found the 'no nonsense, let's get on with it' attitude amongst the general practitioner leaders immensely supportive and helpful. When things got rough I never doubted that I could rely on them.

When the BMA Council met on Wednesday 10 May, it had the BMA's GMC subcommittee's paper on reform of the GMC. It had been produced without any reference to or consultation with the GMC formally, though some BMA members on the GMC had contributed to it because they were members. Jim Johnson introduced the paper with many references to the inefficiencies of the GMC and in particular to the lack of detail on revalidation. Revalidation was the major and underlying issue in the paper. Sam Everington, one of our harshest critics at the last meeting, spoke early. He was keen to make clear that he did not retract in any way from his earlier remarks about the inefficiency of the GMC. However, he went on to say that he supported the direction and the changes that I was attempting to bring about, and felt that any mutterings behind the scenes about my leadership should now be brought out into the open. With that speech the personal critics went to ground.

The paper was severely criticised by many of the BMA Council members themselves. Basically it had the effect of polarising the debate and made it impossible for the BMA Council at that moment to unite around a common position about the future constitution and governance of the GMC.

The GMC Council, 23 and 24 May 2000

The GMC's Council meeting was the next big step in the process. It was to be a testing meeting for the GMC as critical pressure from the BMA of the GMC was continuing to build in advance of the BMA's annual representative meeting in June.

And so to the meeting that had to approve the new drafted consultation paper on revalidation. This paper set out the principles and how revalidation would work in much more detail than hitherto. I had never been to a meeting of the GMC where there were so much foreboding of bad news and with such a poor feel for the expected outcome. Fortunately (and breaking all the rules of political manipulation) the opposition showed their hand immediately. A motion proposed by Sandy Macara and seconded by several other Council members sought to have the publication of the consultation document on revalidation delayed until July. Sandy, in his introduction, spoke of the poor quality of the GMC consultation paper, the high anxiety there was in the profession and the fact that the Council would be making a mistake to publish such an inadequate document at this stage. To do so, he argued, would be to derail the project right at the start.

Several speakers followed for and against, but it soon became clear that GMC members as a whole were getting impatient with what was being seen as a pretty blatant spoiling tactic. Although Jim Appleyard, the Treasurer of the BMA, spoke strongly against revalidation, as did the other signatories to the motion, they were drowned by the other voices. After three-quarters of an hour I asked the Council – with a long list of speakers before me – if they wanted to test the motion, which they did. In the event the amendment to defer publication was lost (those voting for deferment 16, against 68 and with two abstentions).[83] With that, all focused opposition at that meeting to the revalidation consultation document fell away.

Several speakers were very strong on the fact that since this was a consultation paper the people for whom it was intended should have the opportunity to have their say. This included the full range of stake-holders – public, government and employers – as well as the doctors. There was no point, they argued, in polishing the proposals to a point where consultation became meaningless – a *fait accompli*.

In the event this turned out to be one of the most productive Councils ever held. George Alberti, not known as a passionate admirer of the GMC, told me that he thought that it was one of the most effective Councils that he had ever attended.

The Council decided:

- to give the green light to consult on revalidation
- to establish the constitution of the new Interim Orders Committee, giving the GMC greater powers to suspend doctors who may be a danger to the public, pending a full Fitness to Practise investigation
- to approve the appointment of external PCC members, more people to man the hearings and get the waiting times down
- to settle the general principles of the governance of the new GMC
- to approve new ethical guidance on confidentiality.

I was delighted, and relieved, that the GMC had shown more convincingly than ever before that, in the face of strong internal and external opposition, it was capable of developing the reform programme and process of consultation that I had said to Alan Milburn it would do.

The role of the lay members was critical. They were measured, strong on principle, determined yet reasonable. There was no witch-hunting of doctors. But nor was there a willingness to retreat from the principles of good governance that we were all seeking for the sake of unfettered representativeness. They gave the lie to uninformed critics who claimed that the lay members were somehow compliant, ineffective cannon fodder.

Depressingly, the day following the GMC meeting we learnt that there was now to be a vote of no confidence in the GMC at the BMA Senior Hospital Doctors Conference at the month's end. This, presumably, flowed from the failed attempt to derail revalidation – would they never give up and accept the real world?

Ledward again

It was against this background of upheaval and rising fury in the BMA that we had to contend with the publication of the report of the inquiry led by Jean Ritchie QC into the practice of Rodney Ledward, to which I referred earlier.[77] It was published on 1 June, the very day that the BMA consultants were meeting in conference to consider their vote of no confidence in the GMC. If ever there was a case of unfortunate timing, it was this.

I was in Cumbria at the time. I heard on the early BBC news that the GMC was expected to bear the main brunt of the criticism in the Ritchie

Report. I made an early call to Finlay Scott who had heard the same. He had already been on to the BBC to tell them that the line they were taking was at odds with the facts of the Report, the substance of which he had already seen – as indeed so must they. So by lunchtime the reporting had moved its critical focus to the NHS, which more accurately reflected the Report's findings.

Meanwhile, Denis Pereira Gray was at the consultants' meeting. He told me that it was awful. He had spoken, as Vice Chairman of the Academy of Medical Royal Colleges, against the motion of no confidence. The consultants' blood was up and they voted overwhelmingly for the resolution that 'this conference has no confidence in the GMC as currently constituted and functioning'. The dissenting voices, of whom there were five, were mostly leaders of Royal Colleges. Jim Johnson (Chairman, JCC) and Peter Hawker (Chairman, CCSC) did not speak in the debate, nor did Ian Bogle, Chairman of BMA Council. A letter I had sent to Peter Hawker and Jim Johnson, which was intended to be helpful in explaining the reforms and to set a different tone, was not even mentioned. So the doctors present had very partial information.

The press post-mortem on the Ritchie Report on Ledward disappointingly refocused on the GMC again, and we had become the main target. There were critical leaders in *The Times* and in the *Independent*. Encouragingly the government's initial response was supportive of the GMC reforms and revalidation. This suggested that overnight there may have been some kind of reappraisal in government circles that the kind of reform of the culture of medicine would not be accomplishable without the GMC input. If that was right, we reasoned, it would be a plus. Sunday 4 June was not much better. The Sunday papers were critical. The leaders in *The Sunday Times* and the *Independent on Sunday* both called for the abolition of the GMC.

Meanwhile, Denis Pereira Gray told me how very concerned he was about the state of relationships between the BMA consultants' committee and the Academy of the Medical Royal Colleges. Over that weekend I had further conversations with colleagues about the consequences of the BMA consultants' meeting and the likelihood therefore of that translating into a 'no confidence' motion at the forthcoming BMA Annual Representative Meeting. That would be really serious because such a vote would require the BMA Council to act. Interestingly, once again, over that weekend the government had been less overtly hostile to the GMC – indeed, no specific reports other than some neutral reflections by Alan Milburn on the *Breakfast with Frost* programme. But Milburn was firm in that programme on the need not only for new investment in the NHS but for attitudinal change in the NHS, particularly amongst consultants.

Media interest continued apace. On Monday 5 June I had calls from the *Today* programme and BBC television for early morning slots. Then there was Radio 5 Live and, later in the day, Channel 4 news. I felt reasonably comfortable with these interviews. *Hospital Doctor*, on the other hand, was much more hostile. They wanted to know if I was going to resign as President following the consultants' vote. The reporter was very aggressive, particularly when I told him bluntly that the GMC would press on with the programme of reform.

But there was also other news that day. First, I heard that Denis had been elected as Chair of the Academy. This was the first time that the Academy had elected a general practitioner to lead. His performance at the consultants' meeting had confirmed in the minds of many of his colleagues that they had got to have a strong independent advocate. The second piece of news, indicative of the deep division within specialist medicine, was that for the first time in its history the Joint Consultants' Committee had formally split.* The Academy had decided to suspend its membership essentially because of the BMA consultants' attitudes to the GMC's reform programme. Jim Johnson, the JCC Chairman (BMA), was apparently deeply shocked when he was told. The Joint Consultants' Committee had been in existence since 1948, since the Health Service started. It was seen internally and by government as one of the key pillars of the professional establishment, and as such the chasm represented the true extent of the feelings about reform and how these feelings ran so unevenly across the professional tribe.

The Academy then publicly disassociated itself from BMA consultant criticism of the GMC and confirmed its support for the reforms and for my own stance on the matter. It would be misleading to say that the Colleges were ecstatic about revalidation. However, they knew that proper accountability based on regular checks on performance by an independent regulator was essential if public trust in doctors was to be rebuilt. And their leaders showed leadership. They were critical of the GMC about the delays in securing hearings and the inefficiency of its organisation, but their approach was to give support and help to get things right. The contrast with the behaviour of the BMA consultant representatives could not have been more pointed.

So the profession found itself well and truly divided. Ranged alongside the GMC and in support of a firm line on revalidation were the medical Royal Colleges and, as would subsequently become clear very shortly, the General Practitioners' Committee of the BMA. Against were

---

* The Joint Consultants' Committee brings together the standards setting (College) and trade union (BMA) arms of the profession, so that they can speak for specialist medicine as one.

the Central Consultants' and Specialists' Committee of the BMA, the Junior Doctors' Committee and – again to be revealed shortly – the Public Health Committee of the BMA.

Ian Bogle and I met following the consultants' decision, to see what could be done by way of making sure that the representative body in two weeks' time did not make matters worse. A vote of 'no confidence' would be seen outside the profession as the BMA opposing the reforms. He was very anxious. He told me that consultant feelings were running high, particularly against revalidation, but also that their sights were on the inefficiencies of the GMC. I wondered why it had taken them so long to take an interest in the GMC – their help in earlier days to overcome this would have been welcome – and to that he did not reply. I suggested that it would be a good idea if he and his chairmen met with colleagues and myself in the following week. By then we would have the final version of the revalidation consultation document and the five-year review which would map out the extent of the changes to the GMC already achieved. He thought that would be a good idea.

He told me also that he had just come, prior to our lunch, from the Public Health Doctors Conference at the BMA. He had left Sandy Macara haranguing them for about 20 minutes about the iniquities of the GMC, revalidation and myself. So we thought it more than likely that the Conference would follow the BMA hospital consultants' line. We agreed a strong GMC team for the meeting with the BMA. The meeting would be held against the background of continuing adverse criticism in the press of the GMC's handling in the 1980s of the Neale case, which was now being heard by the GMC and of which more in a moment.

In the following few days the politicking continued intensely. The Academy and the general practitioners were doing what they could to mobilise support against a pretty damning resolution of no confidence that was on the agenda of the BMA Conference.

Meanwhile, the business of reform had to go on. Liam Donaldson and I met at Richmond House to talk over the general situation, in particular how the various pieces of the reform jigsaw would come together. We both wondered at the forthcoming BMA meeting whether good sense and good leadership would prevail.

In these roller-coaster times life has its ups and downs. A planned interview for *The Sunday Times* did not go according to plan. An interview intended for the supplement was replaced, without notice to us, by an interview with Lois Rogers, the medical editor, who had a reputation in medical circles for aggressive interviewing. It was one of those profoundly hostile encounters that you know you cannot win. So it was with some trepidation that I left for London on Saturday 17 June, to be ready for an interview with Alistair Stewart on *GMTV* on Sunday morning. I picked up a copy of *The Sunday Times* on the train and my worst fears were realised. I could only speculate what would therefore be in store for me on *GMTV* next morning.

But in fact Alistair was charm itself – he was well briefed on the reform programme that Liam Donaldson and I were pursuing and had heard both of us speak from the same platform recently. I could see the Sunday papers lying on the table in front of him but he never referred to them. Instead, I had what was one of the longest and smoothest interviews throughout the whole of this crisis. As I left the television set Ann Widdecombe, who was coming on, said in passing, 'How did you get away with that?' And he wrote me a charming letter shortly afterwards, wishing us success with the reforms.

Monday saw very good pieces by Sarah Boseley in the *Guardian* and by Nick Timmins in *The Financial Times*. Meanwhile, the high tension now existing between the specialist Royal Colleges and the BMA consultants was showing no signs of lightening. My colleagues and I met with the BMA on 21 June. But first, that day, I had spent a pleasant morning at the presentation of diplomates at the Royal College of Anaesthetists. There was a very good audience. I made the presentation speech that I gathered went down well. But in giving it, I felt strangely disempowered because of the public diminishing of the GMC through its perceived inefficiencies. As its head I felt publicly diminished myself. There was no doubt in my mind that we had sustained heavy damage recently as a result of Shipman, Ledward and now Neale – and the activities of the BMA consultants.

And so to the meeting with the BMA which turned out to be reasonably helpful and good humoured. Peter Hawker began with an apology to me for the conduct of some of his colleagues in personalising the issues in a way that he found unacceptable – this was most helpful in restoring a proper focus to the meeting. Most of the content of his remarks was about revalidation and the consultants' concerns about this. We for our part emphasised that the consultation on which we were about to embark was genuine and that the proper thing for the BMA to do was to make its views known through that. John Chisholm for the general practitioners was firm and positive. Ian Bogle indicated, as the BMA left, that work was continuing behind the scenes to see if the damaging motion calling ultimately for the abolition of the GMC could be ameliorated. Nevertheless, overall our team felt that things had been more positive than they might have been, which was certainly our feeling at our debriefing. And I felt a new spirit of determination abroad amongst many GMC members who were not going to be pushed around by the BMA. In my diary I noted that a new, much more independent-minded regulator was indeed emerging.

The launch of the revalidation consultation: 22 June 2000

We had prepared thoroughly for the revalidation consultation.[84] I had done earlier interviews on the *Today* programme and television. At the press conference proper John Chisholm spoke for general practice, Barry Jackson for specialist medicine and Sue Leggatt as a lay member. Nicola Toynton, a general practitioner, spoke as a working general practitioner. The reporter from *Sky News* was amusing. He kept urging me to answer the questions about the viability of professional self-regulation, and when I got there to his satisfaction he gave me a great smile and thumbs-up sign from behind the camera!

I found the press reaction in all this very interesting. Clearly a good battle within the medical profession was news itself. But talking to people, correspondents were themselves divided into three basic camps – those who were supportive of the GMC reform agenda; those who were against, believing that the GMC should be replaced; and those who did not care and were just after a good story. Journalists are human like everyone else.

On the train home to Newcastle that evening I came across Alan Milburn, travelling alone on his way north. As we met in the compartment his first words were about the BMA meeting and what was going to happen, and whether they would vote for a 'no confidence' motion. We discussed that situation, and more generally, about how the various pieces of his quality agenda and ours could be made to fit together so that the whole system would work better. I emphasised the importance of his making visible the financial underpinning of local clinical governance and proper support for professional development and appraisal – the lessons learnt in general practice training described in Chapter 2. The message I took from listening to doctors around the country at first hand, which I repeated here, was that doctors were not against quality-assured practice. What they objected to was not having the time to do it properly. They wanted to feel valued. A punitive climate was unhelpful, particularly at a time when public opinion was beginning to feel that the consultants as a whole were being punished excessively for the deeds of a few.

This quite informal chat was I felt far more constructive than our last encounter. I sensed that Milburn was up against the reality of an NHS that was faltering, and that he could not repair the damage alone. Part of the solution would require a robust regulator of the medical profession. So in a sense the picture would be of a reformed GMC, strong on doctors' professionalism and the various elements of that – standards, relevant education, regular assessment through revalidation and the removal of those who fail to comply. This would be coupled with strong NHS management, which promoted and supported good practice, and at the same time acted on those dysfunctional practitioners who could be managed and where possible rehabilitated locally, which would be the vast majority.

We spoke about the timetable for GMC reform. I told him that I was going to ask for a special conference in September and, at that time, the aim would be to have a paper on the constitution for consultation. At least the government and the GMC seemed to be going in the same direction.

The BMA Representative meeting

The BMA Representative meeting reached the GMC part of the agenda on Thursday 29 June 2000. As I have indicated earlier, there had been much politicking to try and water down the effects of the no confidence resolution. But, as some of us pointed out, watering down would have little effect if the words 'no confidence' still appeared. The BMA passed the motion on a show of hands by roughly two-thirds to one-third. It stated 'that this meeting, whilst reaffirming its support for self-regulation of the medical profession, had no confidence in the GMC as currently constituted and functioning and calls upon it to initiate urgent reforms of its structures and functions in consultation with the profession'. In the main it was the consultants and hospital doctors who voted for the motion. It was many of the general practitioner leaders who spoke against. The national newspapers were relatively silent. Government was silent. It was the medical press that was in turmoil.

On Monday 3 July I met Alan Milburn on the train again, this time as it neared King's Cross. We had ten minutes or so of conversation. He was anxious about the situation and in particular about the forthcoming GMC Council meeting. Basically the issue was whether the GMC would keep its nerve. By the time I had got to my office his office had already been in touch about a possible meeting.

I had made it clear to him, as I had done in our earlier encounter on the train, that I believed, as did many of my colleagues on the GMC, that the GMC had to win this battle itself for its own integrity, for the public and, indirectly, for the good name and self-respect of the profession. There was nothing that he, at this particular stage, could or should do. This was a matter above all of whether professionally led regulation could be made to work. I felt it was important that he realised that the faction challenging the GMC reform wanted to be able to negotiate with him direct and therefore to regulate standards through contract by the exercise of trade union power. I sensed that he knew this, and I sensed that I was pushing against an open door.*

I felt quite calm at this stage and absolutely determined that the GMC should press on. Many GMC members – both lay and medical – were angry with the BMA and more determined than ever not to be intimidated by them. The core of anti-reformers on the GMC was of course still hard at work with their destabilisation efforts and their demonising of myself. But that's politics – even only medical politics.

In the event Alan Milburn and I met on the evening of Monday 10 July. We were all on our way to a dinner he was giving at the RCP. He was accompanied by his political advisor, Simon Stevens. Finlay Scott and I were there from the GMC. It was a positive and constructive exchange. He was clearly anxious about the relationships with the profession in anticipation of the launch of *The NHS Plan*[66] that was now imminent. He kept coming back again and again to the extent to which the GMC would be prepared to make radical changes to its structure and about the possible timetable. There was some discussion about what it might be most helpful to say about the GMC in *The NHS Plan* and it was left to Simon and Finlay to have a further word about that. It was a good-humoured meeting, and I felt that the GMC's relationships with the government continued to be better than they had been.

The Council tackles governance

A special Council called to get the governance arm of the reforms underway was held on Tuesday 11 and Wednesday 12 July. There were two big issues. One was about future governance – the future size and composition of the GMC. The second was a new think piece on Fitness to Practise, the product of a huge amount of work by members, led skilfully by Douglas Gentleman, and staff led by Isabel Nisbet.

The essential decision was to appoint a group led by Dr Brian Keighley (they worked tremendously hard over the summer) to develop a position on governance on which the GMC could consult.[85] From that preliminary discussion it was already clear that it would not be easy. The question of increasing the lay membership of the GMC was straightforward because all agreed that the current level of 25% was too small. Since the majority favoured a small medical majority on the new Council, in keeping with the principle of professionally led regulation, a provisional figure of 40% lay and 60% medical seemed to be about right.

* William Wells told me later that he had said to Milburn that he thought it essential that the government keep out and that they 'keep their fingers crossed that the GMC wins'.

The real problem was over numbers. The government, many Council members and the Chief Executive wanted a much smaller Council. The consumer bodies thought likewise. The BMA and some of the Colleges were thinking of larger numbers – somewhere around 50 or so – still a significant reduction from the existing position of 104. But the nub was about the size of the controlling body – and whether to be effective in governance really small numbers were required or whether a slightly larger Council with an effective executive would do.

At the least there was an excellent and constructive debate about the issues, a quality of debate that was reflected in consideration of the future Fitness to Practise procedures where quite radical changes were proposed. I shall come back to these later.

At that time I had a conversation with Jim Johnson. Moves were now afoot to restore the relations between the two specialist arms of the profession and bring them together through the JCC. But he was remarkably frank about the BMA vote of no confidence. He confirmed that the argument was all about revalidation. He went further to confirm that what the consultants really wanted was to stick with the contractual arrangements for regulating performance through appraisal – the Borman line – but that they recognised now that revalidation was inevitable. Given this, they wanted as simple and undemanding a process as possible – for instance, just using five summaries of five annual appraisals. They were also concerned, as were general practitioners, about the position of retired doctors who could see that, with revalidation, they might not be able to write prescriptions for their families and friends.

In closing it is important to note this. The BMA vote of 'no confidence' probably damaged the BMA more than it did the GMC, although it did not feel like it at the time. The reason is that the profession was still split. Furthermore, in the outside world one did not have to be deeply perceptive to read the coded messages of resistance to change.

But it could easily have been different. The key determining factor was the decision of the specialist Colleges through the Academy to back the GMC reform, and hold to that. I believe that a completely united specialist body against the GMC could at that time, despite the support for the GMC from general practice, have finished the GMC and professional self-regulation at that point.

But equally had the BMA consultants supported their colleagues in the specialist Colleges, the passage of the reforms would have been far less stormy. Ironically, two years later consultants in England themselves were to lose confidence in that same BMA consultants' committee when they threw out the new contract their negotiators had agreed with the NHS. It seemed that it was the 'unrepresentative' Colleges that were far more in tune with the times. They, like most consultants, had a far better feel for professionalism and the fact that this could not be 'negotiated' as part of a pay deal.

14

Resolution

As I mentioned in the last chapter, the case of Richard Neale was being heard throughout this drama. His case had begun on the 12 June 2000 and ran with breaks until 25 July. It generated huge press comment, much of it seriously critical of past actions by the GMC. The basic facts were these.

Neale, another gynaecologist, came to Britain from Canada, although he was a UK graduate. In Canada he had been struck off the Medical Register following several cases of clinical incompetence between 1980 and 1984. He carried dual Canadian and British registration. In 1985 he sought a post in the NHS. The Canadian authorities had sent two notifications but neither led to action by the GMC. So Neale started to practise at the Friarage Hospital, Northallerton, as a gynaecologist. He finally appeared before the GMC 14 years after he had been struck off in Canada.

At the end of the hearing, Neale was found guilty of all but one of the 35 charges of misconduct laid against him. These charges included performing surgery without having obtained patients' informed consent, modifying surgical procedures such that patients' were put at risk, failing to inform family doctors of complications arising from his incompetence and causing emotional harm to his patients. He was struck off.

I said in a press statement afterwards: 'The case of Richard Neale is shocking and disturbing . . . . I cannot defend the GMC procedures that 15 years ago failed by allowing Richard Neale to practise in this country despite his record in Canada.'

Meanwhile . . .

Meanwhile, the GMC was in close touch with the patient representative and consumer organisations that, not surprisingly, had their own ideas about the constitution of the GMC. There was unquestionably a preference for a lay majority on the new GMC. And there was also a determination amongst them that revalidation should not only be implemented as soon as possible but that it should have proper public involvement and be rigorous. They were far more sceptical than the doctors or NHS managers about the likely consistency and robustness of NHS peer appraisal when it finally got into action.

As with the making of all big changes in life there was much manoeuvring and jockeying for position, and sheer pressure, as the tight deadlines set by the GMC and the government for decision grew nearer.

In the world about there was great activity as the government started to secure support for its new *NHS Plan*. A flurry of consultation papers and proposals for legislation began to flow. The public pressure on the government over the unsatisfactory functioning of the NHS was high and sustained, despite the overwhelming vote of support given in the general election. Indeed the government had now moved the NHS centre stage as a kind of touchstone of its future performance. In this, the modernisation of the regulation of health professionals was only a small part.

At the end of the period the Kennedy Inquiry reported on Bristol.[1] Throughout all the developments that I have been describing the GMC, like the government, had been keeping the Inquiry fully informed of their respective developments. The report fulsomely endorsed the GMC's approach to standards and revalidation.

Within the GMC there was huge activity. The new Interim Orders Committee, which gave the GMC wide powers to suspend doctors under investigation where they appeared to be a threat to patient safety, came into being in August 2000. In addition the GMC now had new powers enabling it to appoint additional people to service Fitness to Practise committees. This was now operational and new members were being trained and started to work on that. A determined effort was being made to crack the backlog problem, not least by hard pressure bearing down on the operating standards that the GMC itself had introduced two years earlier. As part of the modernisation the Education Committee was preparing a new edition of *Tomorrow's Doctors*, designed to imprint the medical curriculum directly onto *Good Medical Practice*. The national examination that the GMC conducted to assess doctors seeking registration from overseas was being completely overhauled. Council members and staff were up to their eyes in the detailed work developing the radically new Fitness to Practise procedures, which were destined to be signed off in November 2002.[86] I have never seen the Council work at such pressure. It is a tribute to so many conscientious people, members and staff alike, that such a powerful forward momentum was sustained in the face of such hostile attitudes from the BMA. It augured well, I thought, for the independent-mindedness that would be required of the GMC in the future.

Last but not least, the negotiations between the government and the consultants and the general practitioners – each separately – on new contracts for both sections of the profession were proving protracted and continued to be so. Resourcing the new commitments to quality where it mattered at the level of individual clinical teams was proving difficult despite the huge amounts of money that the government was now pumping into the NHS.

Finally, things quietened down for the moment after the brush with the BMA – the vote of no confidence dropped like a stone in terms of real impact.

In September 2000 the GMC was host to an international meeting of medical licensing authorities in Oxford. At this meeting the new International Association of Medical Licensing Authorities was launched, following international discussions over the previous two years. This was a success for the GMC because it had played a leading role in getting the new body founded. There was potential for big gains for patients everywhere. It was decided that as an early priority work should start on the development of an international intelligence system and information exchange about doctors on the move from one country to another who had records of professional misconduct or other forms of impaired fitness to practise.

Consent: tensions persist

In the realignment of the public–profession relationship, the issue of consent I mentioned in Chapter 1 was something of a touchstone. It had come to symbolise patient autonomy and the respect people expected from doctors. Two examples now highlighted just how sensitive consent still was.

Retained organs

The first involved the retention of human tissue and organs from children who had undergone post-mortem examination. The issue was retention without parental consent. Cases emerged first in the course of the Kennedy Inquiry and were the subject of a special report. The publicity raised questions elsewhere, especially at the Royal Liverpool Children's Hospital where the practice of a pathologist, Dr Van Veltzen, became the focus of separate inquiry. Van Veltzen was suspended by the GMC pending further investigation. At the time of writing his case has not been heard by the GMC. That notwithstanding, the practices appalled the public, particularly where infants' hearts were concerned. The parents in Liverpool formed an action group, Pity II, through which they channelled their concerns and demands for action.

On 11 January 2001 Liam Donaldson organised a one-day summit on the issue of organ retention at Bristol and the Royal Liverpool Childrens' Hospital, Alder Hey, held as a prelude to the announcement by the government of the results of the Redfern Inquiry into the situation at Alder Hey. Representatives of the parents were invited and there were representatives of the medical profession, hospital management and other parties. I think he had in mind that this kind of occasion would provide for an exchange between doctors – notably pathologists – and parents, and help to defuse what was a very tense situation. He got the idea, he told me, in an earlier visit to Washington where he had seen the technique used in similar circumstances. It was a courageous experiment.

There was a series of carefully controlled presentations that in the event were mainly medical. They revealed a variety of medical attitudes, some of which were perceived as offensive by the parents. There were moving and constructive presentations by parents' representatives.

The dam burst in the afternoon when the discussion was open to the floor and parents were really able to ventilate their feelings and press for legislation to require consent to post-mortem examinations. I was in the audience and found the experience of listening to the thoughts and feelings of those parents quite overwhelming. I was dismayed by the lack of patients' confidence and trust there in the ability or the willingness of the medical profession to handle this itself through professional means.

These feelings were given wider prominence in the way that Alan Milburn chose to herald the release of the report to Parliament. Despite much publicised secrecy surrounding it, he nevertheless broke his own rules and made some pretty hostile comment about doctors in advance of the release day itself. The press reaction, after release, was again hostile because of the conduct of Dr Van Veltzen, the pathologist most involved. A huge nationwide search through all pathology departments in the country ensued. The whole affair had a profound effect on the morale of pathologists, to the point where there was a real danger that paediatric pathological services would collapse. This itself became an issue as it became clear that a section of public opinion thought that pathologists as a group were being treated harshly and unfairly. And there was the question of how medicine could function properly without autopsies to establish causes of death accurately. This story demonstrated the extent to which, in terms of attitude, there were still unresolved cultural differences between patients and doctors, and within the medical profession itself. But it also showed that as the general public came to understand the arguments, there was growing public awareness of, and sympathy for, the complexities of modern practice and the ethical issues with which clinicians had to deal.

Consent and the cancer registries

This dispute was between the government and academic doctors on the one hand, and the GMC and a substantial element of the public on the other. The issue was about whether patients diagnosed as having cancer should have their names put on the appropriate cancer registry for research purposes without their consent. The cancer specialists and the academic community strongly supported the practice that was long established. The registers were important for cancer research. All were agreed on that. So many cancer patients had no idea that information about their condition had been released. An important argument of the researchers was that, if asked, some patients might refuse consent, so damaging the completeness of the database and therefore of future research. However, the GMC in its new 1998 guidance to doctors on consent[87] had stated how important the gaining of consent was. 'Ask the patient' the GMC said. What triggered the reaction was the realisation by doctors who did not seek consent that they exposed themselves to a charge of serious professional misconduct. There had been several conduct cases involving consent issues. So people were aware of the consequences of wilfully disregarding the guidance. Sir Cyril Chantler, Chairman of the Standards Committee, led for the GMC on this. The GMC made the point that the government had a choice. It could either ask Parliament to make cancer a notifiable disease, in which event by authority of Parliament consent would not be needed, or it could improve the anonymisation of the cancer databases so obviating the need for consent.

But hell hath no fury like academics who have their databases challenged! So the GMC found itself at the focus of a considerable row, with the academics and the government on one side, and the GMC and some patients' organisations on the other. It was resolved in the end by the development of a sensible parliamentary process that aimed to secure both equally desirable outcomes. The irony of course is that this was all happening, with the government taking an anti-consent line, at the very same time that it had criticised the pathologists for not getting consent to organ retention. Such were the passions and inconsistencies of the day – a sign of tectonic plates shifting.

The BMA Conference season approaches again

Meanwhile, the Academy and the BMA had come to an agreement on the issue of representation on the new GMC. They wanted a Council of 51 members, of whom 40% would be lay. The position that they were adopting was at odds with the preferred option of the GMC's Governance Working Group that was out for consultation. Their tone was possessive – the GMC was theirs. But the GMC Council itself was quite clear that it had an equal responsibility to its other main stakeholder, the public.

To this end, I and some of my colleagues had a further round of informal discussions with the representatives of patients' organisations, including lay members involved with some of the medical Royal Colleges. They were very clear and determined about their expectations. The public expected to identify GMC registration with good, safe practice. All other matters were secondary to that primary aim. There had to be full public participation. All felt that the proposals on revalidation and for the overhaul of the Fitness to Practise procedures could achieve that provided that they were resolutely and rigorously carried out.

I had a foretaste of the strength of the opposition to the governance proposals when I attended the Council of the BMA on 7 March. The meeting was aggressively hostile, with only one or two speaking in favour of the reforms. Tony Grabham, elder statesman and former GMC member, was the voice of sanity. He urged the BMA to go to war with the government over the new consultants' contract (how prophetic!). At the same time he urged them to talk further with the GMC, which is what they decided to do. So further conversations followed in the weeks into March and April to try and find common ground.

A key meeting was held on Monday 30 April between the representatives of the BMA, the Academy of Medical Royal Colleges and the GMC. We had a strong team that included two lay members, Bob Nicholls and Angela MacPherson, and one of the new young doctors on the Council, Cecilia Bottomley. In trying to find a way forward we raised the possibility of a small Council of about 30 members along the lines proposed by Barry Jackson. But there was impasse. The BMA withdrew at one stage so that they could consider their position privately. They returned to say that although there might be some good ideas as far as they could see as individuals, they were not at all sure that they could put anything forward which would carry their members. I remember vividly how dismayed Angela and Bob were in the face of this intransigence. Cyril Chantler and Graeme Catto (Chair of the GMC Education Committee) were visibly angry.

This confrontational attitude spilled over again at a meeting of the Joint Consultants' Committee to which David Skinner, a GMC official, had gone to answer questions. He had gone at their invitation to discuss some of the detail of the latest consultation papers. He had a very difficult time. Several members had once again vehemently attacked the GMC, revalidation and myself in terms that left David shaken and angry, and as a citizen disgusted with the behaviour that he had witnessed. In retrospect it was a mistake to let David go on his own, unsupported, but no one could do well in such a hostile environment.

It was quite clear, from a conversation I had subsequently with Liam Donaldson, that this incident had provoked concerns about a real split with the GMC. There was the impression that the GMC was not prepared to listen to suggestions about governance and revalidation. It was impossible to say what the position of the government would be in the event that the confrontation persisted. The Kennedy report on Bristol was imminent, and I was aware that, before the end of the year, there were several other serious conduct cases pending that would do nothing to sustain public trust in the profession. It was difficult. The BMA and the Academy had developed a joint position on governance that they wanted to press. But the consumer organisations and the government had different ideas that the GMC had to listen to. It was the kind of tension that was inevitable in searching for a new mechanism that everyone could support. It would mean some concessions all round.

Liam made the helpful suggestion that I might consider adding one further short consultative loop for both revalidation and governance issues, using the kind of summit conference that he had held on Alder Hey. This would bring all the stakeholders together, in public. It would be risky. I thought it over that night and decided to go for it. It might just do the trick.

If it were done it were best done quickly.* I told Finlay Scott and Andrew Ketteringham, the GMC Director of Communications, of my decision on the extra loop. There was consternation. They both thought it would be seen as weakness and as procrastination by us. However, I made it clear that the principles of revalidation were not negotiable. We had consulted enough on that and the more general view of both the profession and the public was very plain. What the conference would do would be to provide the opportunity for the profession's representatives to hear at first hand what the public's representatives and employers were saying. It would provide an opportunity for a clear presentation on revalidation and a further consultation on governance. Most of my colleagues were sceptical. Like Finlay and Andrew, they thought it was a mistake. Sandy Macara thought it was an excellent idea.

Within two days I was in Edinburgh at a meeting of the BMA Council. I think I have never been to such a hostile meeting. I had brought with me the letter inviting the BMA to take part in the proposed stakeholder conference. Some thought that helpful, others saw immediately the possibility of postponing the decision the GMC had to take, to put off the evil day. The usual arguments were rehearsed about the size and representativeness of the GMC. But the real spleen flowed on

---

* *Macbeth*, Act 2.

revalidation. Recent correspondence between the GMC and the BMA on points on which they sought clarification was not sufficient. Someone said, 'Let's get real, this is about jobs.'

It was difficult to stay cool. I said to them that they needed to see the results of the consultation, what other people as well as they themselves thought. I hoped that they would come to the stakeholder conference because they would hear, at first hand, what representatives of the patients' organisations thought about the position. It was no longer a matter of the GMC and the profession deciding these things alone. Those days were over. And I said once again that without a settlement that would be convincing to the public and to government soon, the flow of embarrassing cases would simply reinforce the picture of a profession that was apparently incapable of managing its own affairs.

But in spite of this, in the run-up to the GMC Council in May criticism of revalidation continued. Disappointingly, some members of the BMA had decided also that, in addition to harrying the GMC, they would harry me personally at every point for the remainder of my presidency. There was a move within the Council, led by Ed Borman, to institute a vote of no confidence in myself. I consulted about that with colleagues over the weekend, in one of my well-known telephone consultation ring rounds, and it was pretty clear that such a vote would be well defeated, if ever called. But in the next day or two I thought very carefully about the position and talked it through with my wife. My presidency was entering that dangerous stage when, within 12 months of its natural end, I could become a lame duck, especially in the face of sustained opposition, which could unseat the whole reform programme. I was quite clear that I needed to see the programme through but the timetable for that took us to the end of the year. Then the Council would have either got agreement amongst the stakeholders on all aspects of the reform programme or would not, and the government would have to step in. What I needed to do was to be absolutely strong – untouchable – for the next six months until the end of the year.

Unwittingly my critics made it easy for me. On the morning of the Council Ed Borman told Finlay Scott that he would not now be putting his motion of no confidence because he and his supporters had decided 'to give the President and the GMC one more chance'. That decided me. I would announce that I would step down in the February of the following year, six months before the absolute limit of my final term of office. But I would do that only after the vote seeking legislation for revalidation was out of the way. In this way I would remain politically as strong as possible to get the governance and Fitness to Practise reforms through – the rest of the reform package.

It was an attractive idea. Securing agreement on the reforms would, for me, represent the completion of my objective when I was elected. The policy package would be complete. The GMC would then need to go into implementation mode. It was a natural breakpoint for a change of president who could carry the momentum on implementation forward to the point where the 'old' GMC would be replaced by the 'new' GMC.

The general mood of the Council was to get on and seek legislation – the view that the revalidation proposals were not sufficiently well developed was simply not accepted. There were the usual delaying tactics, with which we were by now all familiar. It was Sandy Macara who proposed an amendment to the motion to the effect that there would be consultation on the next stages before revalidation was actually implemented. With that amendment he provided a fig leaf for the opposition for, of course, by law there would have to be consultation anyway. So the final motion was carried by 77 votes to two, with one abstention.[88] Everybody felt good, a decisive win.

Plain sailing from now on

Immediately after the Council I met George Alberti, Barry Jackson and Jim Johnson to see what further could be done, prior to the stakeholder conference, to get an agreement on the governance issue. We returned to the Royal College of Surgeons' proposal for a Council of around 30. We agreed amongst ourselves that a Council of 35 might be acceptable to the GMC, assuming it was acceptable elsewhere in the profession. It might also be acceptable to the lay stakeholders. The others dispersed to a meeting of the Joint Consultants' Committee where that line was endorsed. And that became the position that the BMA and the Colleges would speak to at the stakeholders' conference. I had informal talks with the patient organisations that wanted an even smaller body. But they recognised too that they could come together around the sort of size that had emerged.

In the event the stakeholders' conference was successful. Chaired very effectively by Alistair Stewart, the television presenter, it allowed each of the principal stakeholders to hear what the others had to say – in public, on the record. The Council met again in July and endorsed the proposals without much ado. Later, in November, it settled the main framework for the third arm of reform, that of Fitness to Practise, in a manner along lines that seemed to satisfy both the profession and the public stakeholders. Government did not comment at that stage although considerable informal discussion had suggested that it would accept this line also.

So all three limbs of reform were now in place – revalidation, Fitness to Practise reforms and a new GMC. The new GMC will be fundamentally different from the old. The GMC had ended the longstanding perception of ambivalence about its primary purpose. From now on its basic job was to protect patients by making sure that they were looked after by competent, honest doctors. It was not there to 'represent' doctors – that was for others to do. It strongly endorsed the principle of self-regulation for individual doctors, extending the principle to the notion of collective self-regulation in clinical teams. It adopted the concept of professionally led regulation for the whole profession based on partnership with the public. And it reinforced the fact that it is licensure that must provide the public with the ultimate guarantees about the fitness of their doctors to practise medicine to an agreed standard anywhere in the UK.

At the meeting of the Council in November 2002, Professor Sir Graeme Catto was elected President. He took over from me on 1 February 2003.

15

The doctors' tale: the next chapter

In January 2001 I gave the Lloyd Roberts Lecture at the Royal Society of Medicine.[60] In that lecture I summarised the story I have just told – a story that is uncomfortable for doctors. I believed then, and still do, that the profession collectively had to confront its past – and to learn from that – in order to move forward to deliver its best in a modern way in today's world. Not surprisingly the reactions to the lecture were divided. For the public and the press the message represented a state of affairs with which lay people could readily identify. Furthermore, the significance of the message lay in the fact that it came from within the profession. The response from the profession was mixed. Many doctors reacted positively because they already knew in their hearts that change was not only inevitable but also right. On the other hand some doctors objected strongly. They took it, wrongly, as personal criticism.

In the last two years I have found that some in the profession have still not fully accepted the hard facts of life. Effective relationships with patients and quality care are already a reality for many. Yet if we were fully to acknowledge what was not right as well as taking appropriate credit for what the profession has done well, the public would believe more easily that the profession is determined, collectively, to ensure that very shortly this standard will be extended to all. The new regulatory framework is now in place for that change to happen. But for patients and the morale and self-respect of the profession itself, it is doctors in their hearts, minds and attitudes that will make the difference at the final count between excellent and just acceptable medical care.

In this chapter I reflect on what I think are important lessons from the story and look to some implications for the future. These views are entirely personal. But they are consequential to the story, and are very much influenced by my own experiences over the years.

Looking back

The medical culture

Looking back on this era of medical history, the main themes have revolved around my central belief that culture matters more than anything else. For good or ill the medical culture has dictated the profession's behaviour and its responses to external forces. Throughout this period we have seen its effects, expressed in individual attitudes to patients, working colleagues and working practices, and collectively in the various expressions of tribalism and attitudes to professional regulation. Overwhelmingly the medical culture has been, and still is, founded on the fact that the majority of doctors want to do their best for their patients, and that best has been, and still is, frequently at the expense of a doctor's own interests and personal needs. The dedication, skill and commitment of most doctors in the UK are too often taken for granted, yet they are amongst the most important weapons society has in the fight against disease and pain.

Professional culture expresses and reflects professional values and standards as well as societal expectations and mores that exist at any one time. What my tale shows is that in recent years the medical culture in some important respects has not kept pace with changing societal values and expectations. As the gap has widened so conflict became inevitable. I profoundly regret that for some patients their experience of medical care ended in tragedy before the tectonic plates shifted sufficiently. Moreover, some of us who were in a position to make a difference sadly were not able to persuade and influence soon enough and effectively enough to prevent at least some of their pain and suffering.

Having said that, doctors do not work in isolation. Their culture is shaped by and dependent on the structure, policies and culture of the organisations in which and for which they work. For the last half century that in effect has meant the NHS because the private sector has been relatively small. The story I have told shows that there have been real problems of collusion between successive governments and the medical profession because both had direct responsibilities for the delivery of medical care. It was sometimes explicit but more often unspoken. The collusive relationship began at a time when across the country, in all walks of life, the producer was king, and customers – including patients – were expected to be grateful, passive and uncritical. Patients and the public had very little say.

A major underlying cause, as I showed in Chapters 3 and 5, lay in the trade-offs between governments seeking to limit expenditure on healthcare and the profession seeking to retain maximum clinical autonomy.

Not surprisingly, therefore, there were times when collusive behaviour worked against the public. For me, the most striking example, which goes right to the heart of the patient safety issue, was the toleration by both the profession and successive governments of the large tail of poor or unacceptable general practice in the 1950s right through to the late 1990s. The result was that thousands of people registered with poorly performing doctors were put at completely avoidable risk. I belonged to the minority group, largely members of the RCGP, that tried to do something about it. We knew at first hand just what resistances and tensions resulted from going against the institutional tolerance of poor practice. We knew how it felt to 'break ranks' with the general culture of protectionism within the profession reflected in earlier times in general practice by the powerful General Medical Services Committee of the BMA. I hope that some feel for the flavour of that conflict has come through in the story. But there were other examples of undesirable collusion. These included the exploitation of too many of the doctors who came to work in this country from overseas, the turning of a blind eye to critical clinical standards issues at times of doctor shortage, the inordinate time taken to modernise basic medical education and specialist training, the unsatisfactory local arrangements for investigating complaints about poor clinical care in hospital consultants and the slowness of both the state and the doctors to put quality in healthcare nearer the top of the agenda.

Collusive behaviour extended to the regulation of doctors. It was this, primarily, which caused both professional self-regulation and professional regulation by the state through employment contracts to fail. The self-interest of the profession and of successive governments, when coupled with the fact that service provision and regulation in the NHS were too closely bound together, made it almost impossible to ensure that the public interest would always come first. The absence of significant systematic public/patient input – other than through grossly under-resourced Community Health Councils – virtually guaranteed that.

Thus the GMC was whatever the big players wanted it to be. This does not absolve it from responsibility for its failings. But either the government or the profession could have changed it much earlier had they been really determined and taken their responsibilities as stakeholders seriously. However, as we have seen, they were more interested in managing the performance of doctors through contracts of employment or contracts of service that they controlled themselves. This professional regulation by contract did not protect patients effectively from poorly performing doctors. Hence the frustration of the public who had no serious independent say in the hospital NHS complaints machinery and who thought that the GMC, as the statutory regulator for all doctors, was biased against them.

Bristol

The true significance of Bristol and the other high-profile failures is that it signalled the moment when change became inevitable. I have shown that both successive governments and the profession had already started to change course in the years preceding Bristol – but not quickly or far enough. In response to Bristol the GMC, now strongly supported by general practice – both RCGP and BMA – and by the specialist medical Royal Colleges, led the change from within towards the new culture of professionalism which welcomed the principle of patient autonomy. The government set about its own extensive modernisation plans. The last stand of those in the medical profession who were against new ideas on credible professional accountability came via the Central Consultants' and Specialists' Committee of the BMA. Revalidation was their battle-ground. In their negotiations with the Department of Health about appraisal, which feeds into revalidation for most doctors, it seems they still hankered after the old collusive relationship. They seemed keen to keep the evidence needed to demonstrate good practice to the absolute minimum. Hence the major cause of conflict with the GMC, which wanted robust evidence of performance, an equally robust appraisal process and direct public involvement. But that stage is passing. As the dust settles, I hope we will look back to find that the dramatic transition from one professional culture of medicine to another new one was actually achieved with relatively little trauma.

One reason for that lack of trauma lies in general practice where the culture change had been underway for some time. As I look back, I see the significance of the ferment in general practice in the early 1970s more clearly now than I saw it then. In the new vocational training there were all the roots of the new professionalism – positive patient orientation, explicit standards, a regulatory framework for ensuring compliance, focus on behaviour and communication, the professionalisation of teaching, serious professional development and so on. That movement in a section of general practice, led throughout by the RCGP, established the value of seeking a positive demonstration of good practice in its own right, as well as a counter to the challenge of poor practice. And that is the basis of revalidation.

Another reason is the vigour with which specialist medicine through the medical Royal Colleges and specialist societies reacted after Bristol. For example, the surgical colleges, the anaesthetists, the obstetricians and gynaecologists, and the radiologists got down to clinical governance and revalidation in a positive and serious way. The heart surgeons in particular, through the Society of Cardiothoracic Surgeons of Great Britain and Ireland, really began to show what could be done in defining and assessing surgical practice.

Leadership

Lastly the theme of leadership has permeated this story. In the medical profession it has been essentially reactive and badly co-ordinated. Over the years there has been no effective collective leadership determined to make sure that professional regulation worked properly. In the recent conflict it would be easy to demonise the BMA. But the BMA was itself divided. As I have said, the BMA's powerful consultants' committee was the main focus of opposition to meaningful change. But the current leadership of general practice in the BMA was fully persuaded of the need for serious change, and acted accordingly. Critically the leaders of all the medical Royal Colleges, co-ordinated through the Academy of Medical Royal Colleges, demonstrated throughout the recent crisis that they not only recognised the need for change but also were prepared to work hard with the GMC to achieve it. They started to lead effectively together and that leadership was decisive. As in all walks of life, leadership is a critical ingredient in managing change successfully.

These, then, are some of the general lessons from which we must learn.

Looking ahead

As we look to the future we can be sure that the pace of scientific discovery and technological development in medicine will continue. For patients this is basically good news in terms of improvements in diagnosis and treatment, and better outcomes reflected in a better quality of life. Equally, we can be sure that attitudes to health and healthcare will evolve. As patients and consumers of healthcare we will become far better informed, take much more responsibility for our own care and exercise more choice and influence as to who will look after us, how we will be treated, where and when.

It is the information age as much as medical science that is driving change. As a result, the globalisation of medical practice has already begun. It is the hi-tech, interventionist specialities such as transplant and cardiac surgery that are leading the way as specified outcomes and risks for specified procedures are being established and made publicly available for all to see. On the Internet and in our newspapers we can expect more international, publicly accessible information in future on clinical and professional standards, and comparative data about the clinical performance of individual doctors, clinical teams and healthcare institutions, and of patients' experiences of them. The work of the Picker Institute, Europe in systemising and publishing comparative information about patient experiences, and the publication of performance information by government agencies such as CHAI and the Audit Commission, and by private independents like Dr Foster, give a foretaste of what is to come. Consumer and patient groups are contributing to these developments, helping to drive them. The Internet has just as surely transformed their connections and communications about health-care worldwide, and therefore their growing ability to influence the performance and practices of clinicians.

This is the changing context in which we have to view the future provision, organisation and regulation of healthcare now. And this is the context in which we need to look at some of the main lessons from the past, and what we might do differently in future as a result.

At the beginning of the book I said that as patients we want three things. We want good access to care when needed; we want competent, honest health professionals who will treat us with respect, kindness and courtesy; and we want care by a clinical team we know we can rely on to give us optimum quality and safety. These are the fundamentals. Access is about the capacity of the healthcare system. This is an important subject in its own right, which is at the forefront of the political debate today. I have nothing to add here, save to say that in the UK today it is manifestly insufficient. The government knows that, and is trying to correct the deficiencies.

However, to achieve the other two requirements that are essentially about quality, I believe that several key changes must happen soon. The fact of the arrival of the autonomous patient needs to be fully recognised and with it full acceptance of the importance of patient choice; some fundamental changes to the NHS; a new approach to professionalism in all the health professions and fully independent professional and institutional regulation. More needs to be done in all these areas if the expectations of the public and the health professions are to be fully realised.

The autonomous patient

In the story I have described the rise of the citizen as an autonomous patient and the end of unquestioning deference to doctor or the system. The very fact that every citizen can, through the Internet, access the whole of the knowledge base of medicine without the consent of, or prior interpretation by, doctors is in itself a statement of the magnitude of the power shift which is still taking place. This change in the balance will result in a more adult relationship between patient and doctor, public and profession.

In the empowerment of patients, choice is fundamental. It can have powerful beneficial effects such as, for example, strengthening the doctor–patient relationship by enhancing the doctor's sense of account-ability to the patient. Yet in the NHS choice has been relatively limited hitherto. This has been due partly to the fact that in the UK throughout the life of the NHS there has been a strongly egalitarian approach – the welfare state. As a nation we have prized equity of access and provision above all – everybody must have the same. It has brought huge benefits, even though in practice the distribution and quality have often been far from equitable.

There is today a shift from egalitarianism to personal autonomy in all walks of life. Healthcare is no exception. In real life, when we are confronted with serious illness in the family, we want to do what we think is best for our loved ones. We put equity to one side to try and get the best doctor, the best treatment. We exercise choice if we can. The pressure to broaden the scope for choice is bound to increase as more and more people feel they should have that opportunity, particularly as they gain access to more and better information about the technical performance of individual doctors and the results of clinical care in individual hospital units and general practices. That will be their starting point for making informed decisions. This trend carries with it huge consequences for the quality, provision and organisation of health services, for regulation, and for the culture of professionalism – across all health professionals and managers – on which, in terms of quality, so much will depend. And it has equally profound implications for our responsibilities as citizens to those people who have the same individual right to choice, but who for economic or other reasons are least able to exercise it. Because the trend towards more choice is unstoppable there is an urgent need now for a serious public debate and examination of the subject and all its ramifications.

A National Health System?

The second area where change is needed is in the organisation of our health services. I have been a lifelong supporter of the NHS. Overall I think it has served us well, particularly in the provision of well-distributed, increasingly well-organised primary care and in the hospitals responding to the needs of the acutely ill. However, we have now outgrown the existing NHS model. A much-loved punchball alternately praised and vilified by the British people, it has become a relic of an era of centralised state control and provision that is passing. We see it even today in producer mode, as an institution, as an end in itself in which the provision of care and regulation are still too closely intertwined. The NHS has low expectations of its performance because, being centrally driven and controlled, the opportunities for organisational innovation and individual professional initiative and development are limited and inevitably will remain so. It still scrimps on quality. Given that as a country we aspire to be an international leader in healthcare, this is not a sustainable position either for the patients who use the NHS or for the practice and morale of people who work in it.

We need to discard this centralised bureaucratic strait-jacket. We need a more flexible system of healthcare whose only purpose is to serve people in need and which will meet the expectations of the autonomous patient. We might be helped in this if we stop thinking about a National Health Service as a rather rigid institution – and start thinking about a National Healthcare System (still NHS!) embracing a diverse range of services and providers – public, 'not-for- profit independent' and private. We must retain the basic values that are important to us, but free up our thinking about how practically to achieve much more diverse provision of care – public and private – and therefore secure the much needed clearer separation between the providers of healthcare and systems of regulation. Diverse provision should be far more responsive to personal needs and to the needs of local communities. We need to promote more choice as well as respond to pressures for it. Diverse provision, when coupled with truly independent regulation, would severely limit the opportunities for the kind of collusive relationship between government and profession that I have shown has been so damaging in and to the NHS in the past. And the new National Healthcare System would gain from those employed and contracted within it a commitment, confidence and empowerment, not to the organisation but directly to their patients.

Despite the experiments with NHS trusts, and now Foundation Hospitals, I do not see how a serious diversification of provision and truly independent regulation will ever be achieved, without a change at the top of our health service. In England and Wales the Secretary of State for Health and his or her Ministers function primarily as the Chair and executive board members of the NHS, the provider organisation of most but not all of the country's healthcare. There are similar arrangements elsewhere in the Kingdom. We need to end this situation. As a nation we place an impossible burden on Ministers, whatever their political persuasion. Their current roles and responsibilities include securing optimal standards of practice and care through regulation, helping us as a nation decide what healthcare we can afford, and particularly managing the operational practicalities of the NHS today. We expect them to reconcile the huge conflicts of interest between these, as well as fighting to survive the pressures of political ambition and success. It is mission impossible. Other countries with more successful systems than ours do not constrain themselves in this way. Now our political leaders need to free up the structural block at the top of the system as soon as possible. The liberating effect of that itself would symbolise the seriousness of their intent and dynamise change.

My proposal is, therefore, that we need Ministers of the Crown to leave the business of managing healthcare provision to others, unconnected directly with government, who can give it their undivided attention and commitment. The organisation and management of healthcare should not be a function of politicians. On the other hand the government's real responsibilities, which will always be political, are concerned with resolving the big strategic issues in health. Ministers need to concentrate on, for example, how we should pay for healthcare, what we are prepared to afford, and how we reconcile individual choice with the need to protect those who are less able to look after themselves. They need to be looking beyond the provision of healthcare, to the much bigger picture of the public health itself and how we are to become a healthier nation. They should be leading the debate about these important issues of public policy, ethics and strategy, with Parliament setting the parameters and framework within which the providers function. In that scenario Ministers would unequivocally be on the side of the patients and the regulators, not the providers. And the health professionals in the hospitals and primary care – the providers – would have much more freedom to deliver the services required of them in ways they think will give the best outcomes both for patients and themselves.

The new professionalism

And so to the third area for the future which is about the health professions. As must be abundantly clear by now, I regard professionalism as the key to the future relationship between practitioners, public and the employers.

But here I confine myself to doctors. A key lesson from this story is how lightly, almost dismissively, some doctors have regarded their professionalism in the past. They have used the word without really analysing and understanding its true significance. True professionalism embodies not only values and standards, but also the determination to see these are practised in full by individuals and the profession collectively.

In future as doctors we must take our professionalism – and with it professional regulation – more seriously, to see this as our basic professional asset, to be nurtured, researched, developed, taught and protected as medical practice continues to evolve. We need to see professionalism as a living thing, the contemporary embodiment of the medical culture – not as a dry ethical concept.

A fundamental breakthrough came when the GMC abandoned virtually unrestricted autonomy for individual doctors in favour of a clear set of principles, *Good Medical Practice,* and the linking of compliance with those principles to a doctor's continuing registration. The principles – essentially a code – founded and maintained on a consensus derived from full public involvement, represent a definitive statement of what both the public and the medical profession expect of their doctors at any point in time. They are a statement of doctors' duties and responsibilities that go with their rights and privileges. In other words they are the essence of the profession's side of the regulative bargain between public and profession.

So how does the new professionalism differ from the old? It starts by recognising the importance of the autonomous patient. A sound ethical foundation, scientific and technical competence, the interests of the patient and the notion of service are still fundamental core values. However, it embraces now evidence-based medicine rather than clinical pragmatism, the recognition of the importance of attitudes and behaviour, partnerships with patients, and accountability rather than personal autonomy. At the same time, the new professionalism is about teamwork rather than individualism, collective as well as personal responsibility, transparency rather than secrecy, empathetic communication and above all of respect for others. An unreserved commitment to quality improvement through clinical governance is fundamental. The profession of medicine must become, as Freidson[89] said, 'enthused with a spirit of openness, driven by the conviction that one's decisions must be routinely open to inspection and evaluation, like the openness that pervades science and scholarship'.

In implementing the new professionalism, the lessons from the early years of training trainers in general practice are important to recall, because they worked. As I showed earlier, the keys lay in professional leadership, role modelling and the whole panoply of methods used to aid serious professional development.

New thinking about professionalism means rethinking our medical institutions – the medical Royal Colleges, the professional societies and the BMA. Now that the direction of travel is clear they have a unique opportunity – indeed I would say an obligation – to rethink their purpose, functions and organisations in ways that, individually and together, will help to cement the partnership and secure the new settlement between the profession and the public.

The medical Royal Colleges and the professional societies working closely with the universities can become the front-line leaders in embedding the new professionalism in practice and education. Their authority and influence would be immensely strengthened were their memberships and fellowships to become clearly and directly linked in future with ongoing excellence in practice, as the RCGP has done with its Fellowship by Assessment. Revalidation would then be an effective but very light touch. The Academy of Medical Royal Colleges, already speaking with more authority, could develop as the collective public voice of the profession on standards in each branch of the profession.

The BMA is approaching a crossroads. If healthcare does indeed diversify, the role of the BMA as a single professional representative voice on conditions of service will inevitably change. Signs of this were already beginning to be seen following the results of the ballot for the proposed consultants' contract in the UK in 2002. Some would see this loss of traditional trade union bargaining power as a threat. But the new world could offer the BMA, as a professional society, a real opportunity to reposition itself, not least to establish modern medical professionalism in society's mind as an indispensable asset for patients as well as doctors. Complementing the work of the Royal Colleges and the GMC, it could, to give just one example, engage the public directly in helping to secure the practising environment and working conditions for doctors necessary to make quality a reality for all. This has become urgent for patients as well as the clinicians who are exposed to constant pressure to do more, which they feel is at the expense of quality. The present situation in the NHS is untenable, the product of compromise and the British habit of 'muddling through'. New thinking is needed.

A more confident, more assertive profession, working with and for the public, should play a more influential and proactive role in shaping the future direction of medicine, explaining the limits as well as potential. The notion of the profession accepting a civic duty of this kind would of itself contribute to the further building of public confidence and trust. If we follow this kind of holistic road to professionalism the public and the profession together could revolutionise the practice of medicine. Britain would not be alone. This kind of thinking is being explored and developed elsewhere, in particular in Canada, the USA and Australasia.

Independent regulation

The story has demonstrated why regulation in future needs to be robustly independent of any sectional interest. The combination of rigorous regulation, good clinical governance and the ability of patients to make well-informed choices about their doctors and hospitals offers the best way of assuring quality in future. It will provide a powerful incentive for individual health professionals to be sure of their competence in the widest sense, and for clinical teams and institutions to be sure that they have effective clinical governance.

The new or reconstituted regulators for the health professions and institutions are already coming into action, and it is certainly the stated intention of Parliament that they should indeed be 'independent' of but accountable to it. However, I question whether sufficient thought has been given as to how that might best be done. In my Lloyd Roberts lecture[60] I said that we need a mechanism that gives the public direct access, through Parliament, between the citizen and the regulators taking decisions on their behalf. We need Parliament to think imaginatively about how this might best be done, what might be an improvement on the existing Select Committee arrangements. The MP Frank Field and I have already suggested an all-party committee, drawn from both Houses, which would be well supported administratively. The model of the US Senate Hearings came to mind. That would be one way – there will be others. Whichever method emerges, accountability would flow from the information the regulators would be required to make available publicly about their stewardship of their part of the regulatory system. This openness would be enhanced by the public and press scrutiny of the results that would be an inherent part of the process. The Secretary of State for Health, freed from provider responsibilities as I have suggested, should lead and co-ordinate on behalf of the government, Parliament and the nation.

The role of the Council for the Regulation of Health Care Professionals (CRHP) has yet to be clarified in practice. There is certainly an important co-ordinating function to be carried out between all the regulators of the individual health professions, such as the GMC and the reconstructed General Dental Council. The purpose of this body is to do that. But in addition there should be consistency of values and standards, and sharing of methodologies and processes across all the healthcare regulators whenever that is appropriate. But the most valuable thing the new Council could do would be to help to develop and embed the principles of the new professionalism in all the health professions. That way lies the best chance of achieving cultural change. What it must not do regularly is to interfere with the direct accountability of the regulator of each profession directly to Parliament itself. It is those regulators, not intermediaries or any co-ordinating mechanism, that actually make the decisions that will affect patients. Parliament has to be able to question them directly.

Those with a passion for simplification have argued that the CRHP could itself become the single regulator of the health professions, with each of the health professions represented through the current Councils that would become branch offices. That approach – one size fits all – would be administratively tidy. But such tidiness should never be allowed to erode the fundamental importance of a profession feeling a true sense of pride in and ownership of its culture embodied in its professional standards.

The same principles should apply incidentally to the new institutional regulators such as CHAI and the Audit Commission. I agree with Sir Ian

Kennedy's recommendation[1] that in future CHAI's most important function should be to validate, and revalidate, institutional quality. I believe that this should be done at the level of the individual hospital unit or primary care team. That is where it matters practically to patients. That is the level at which patients want to be sure that the service they are about to use – be it a general practice or a particular hospital speciality unit – is of the required standard. That is the level at which they have to make choices. Hospital league tables, star ratings and so on should then all be dispensed with, to the benefit and relief of all.

The new GMC

So what properties and qualities should we look for in the regulator of a health profession now? Rudolph Klein[72] underlined the interdependence of public policy and professional regulation when he said: 'The aim of public policy is to make the medical profession accountable for its performance. The aim of professional regulation is to make individual practitioners more accountable to their peers. The success of the former strategy depends crucially on the latter, on instituting professional regulation at the local level (personal self-regulation and clinical governance). The precise balance between the two will depend on the extent to which the medical profession can be trusted to honour its part of the bargain.'

The new GMC should become a role model of good regulatory practice and governance. It will be very different, not least because of the much more even balance between public and professional membership. It must be, as Cyril Chantler has put it, the keeper of the medical profession's conscience through its ultimate stewardship of the profession's standards.

Standard setting is the starting point – both standards of practice and of medical education. *Good Medical Practice* provides the clear and accepted basis and the GMC needs to keep this under review. Equally, we should expect the GMC vigorously to develop and co-ordinate all stages of medical education, in partnership with the universities and medical Royal Colleges, so that the standards of education properly reflect the standards of practice that are required.

Registration remains the core function. Clarity about good medical practice must lead to more clarity about the criteria for joining the Medical Register initially. One clear principle must be established – at the point of the grant of full registration, the same criteria and competencies should apply regardless of whether a doctor has trained in the UK or in any other country. Methods for assessing compliance need to be further adapted and synchronised to meet this requirement. Some will point to legal constraints guaranteeing the free movement of doctors in

Europe that would make it difficult. But we should not hide behind the law. We should be clear about the right thing to do, and then find out how to overcome legal hurdles – even starting the slow process of knocking them down where necessary.

Equally, clarity about the basis of good practice should lead to more clarity about significant departures from it. As I see it, the impairment of fitness to practise and the sanctions that should apply should in future be essentially standards issues. It will be the job of the Fitness to Practise panels, now suitably separated from the policy arm of the GMC, and which already may have lay chairs and an appropriate balance of lay and professional members, to investigate, prosecute and decide in individual cases of breach against the policy template provided by the GMC. This sort of arrangement would be analogous to the relationship between Parliament making the law and the various agencies – including the courts applying the law in individual cases.

The use of explicit professional standards will require the future GMC to develop even more expertise in the assessment of doctors' competence and fitness to practise at all points where registration is involved. Whether it does assessments itself or delegates or shares the responsibility with others – and it does and will continue to do both – assessment against standards has to become the GMC's prime business method because it underpins registration and the granting of licenses to practise. It will mean more collaboration with the universities, the medical Royal Colleges and any others who share these responsibilities.

The real test of the trustworthiness of the new GMC will be the credibility of the standards of competence, care and conduct it sets for revalidation and the robustness of the evidence it is prepared to accept from doctors to demonstrate their compliance. Public involvement in the processes will be essential. In fact, most doctors will offer evidence derived from local clinical governance and appraisal. This could be highly variable. Consequently public and professional confidence will be determined largely by the effectiveness of the regular quality checks that the GMC will use to show that revalidation is sound, reliable and consistent. CHAI will be able to contribute to these checks from its perspective where it has jurisdiction. But at the end of the day the buck stops with the GMC – the licensing authority. It alone is ultimately responsible for ensuring that the doctors it has licensed to practice are indeed practising in accordance with the standards it says are necessary.

And lastly . . .

Looking back over the last 50 years we can see much more clearly now that we have been living through a hugely significant change in the doctor–patient–society relationship. The concepts of patient autonomy and of partnership between public and profession now embody a far greater awareness of patients' needs and expectations. In bringing this closer to fruition, the patients' stories and experiences – the Bristol and Alder Hey parents, Shipman's victims, the women damaged by Ledward and Neale, and the others – have all given focus for my colleagues and myself. For us as doctors, our understanding of the new relationship with our patients and the public finds its outward expression in the values and standards of the new medical culture, the new professionalism.

Postscript

The new GMC

The model

The new GMC that emerged retained the basic functions of the old in respect of professional standard setting, education, registration and fitness to practise, but with substantial differences in its ethos, governance, Fitness to Practise procedures and the new function of revalidation.

The model that the GMC evolved to encapsulate these fundamental changes was based on the following:

- an ethos that puts the interests of patients at the heart of everything the GMC does
- an explicit code of duties and basic standards of practice – *Good Medical Practice* – agreed as desirable in a doctor by all stakeholders
- the direct linkage of *Good Medical Practice* with doctors' registration to ensure compliance
- robust measures to make sure that those joining the Register have the qualities that are expected, that those on the Register continue to practise in accordance with them and that doctors who fail to comply are disciplined and if necessary removed from the Register
- the embedding of the professional standards into medical education so that the system is capable of producing doctors who have the agreed qualities
- the embedding of the standards, either directly or indirectly, into doctors' contracts of employment so that a linkage is established with employers' local systems of clinical governance.

The GMC itself is to have a new structure and new arrangements for governance, based on a partnership between doctors and the public. It will be fully accountable to Parliament. It meets the basic requirements of a professional regulator defined by the National Consumer Council.

The model was the basis for consultation with all stakeholders. Those consultations were concluded successfully in November 2001. It was endorsed by the Kennedy Report in July 2001. In May 2002 the government published a draft Order for the New GMC, based on the final recommendations put forward by the GMC. In December 2002 the new statutory framework was implemented by Parliament.

The essential elements of the new framework are set out below.

Structure and governance

The new GMC will be a small strategic organisation with a membership of no more than 35. There will be a majority of medical members (including two appointed by the medical schools and medical Royal Colleges). Lay members will constitute about 40% of the Council. The Council will be led by a medically qualified President. It will be founded on the principles of effectiveness, inclusiveness, transparency and accountability.

The government had set out its expectations of the New GMC in the paper supporting the draft Order. It said it should:

- be smaller and more strategic
- give priority to patients' interests
- have clear and effective mechanisms for accountability
- be responsive to change and health service needs
- adhere to the criterion for a modern regulatory body set out in *Supporting Doctors, Protecting Patients*
- be positioned for a quick intervention when public protection is needed.

This list conformed to the public and the professions' expectations of a revised body.

Revalidation

Revalidation as described earlier is the process through which doctors must be able to demonstrate on a regular basis that they remain fit to practise because they continue to comply with *Good Medical Practice* that describes the duties and responsibilities of a good doctor. It places on the individual doctor the onus to prove continuing fitness to hold a licence to practise, rather than as now placing the onus on the GMC to prove unfitness. Revalidation is based on the positive affirmation of good practice rather than the negative identification of 'bad apples.'

Currently, any doctor who holds any category of GMC registration may apply for a licence. In future the rights and privileges currently attaching to registration (such as prescribing drugs and other professional functions) will be transferred to the licence to practise. Doctors who do not revalidate will not hold a licence to practise and therefore will not be able to prescribe drugs or practise clinically.

The key to securing revalidation lies in the evidence offered by the doctor of professional performance. Revalidation will be granted on the basis of assessments made of evidence of the doctor's performance against the principles of *Good Medical Practice*. For the vast majority of doctors who are in employment – which includes all NHS medical staff – annual appraisal should encompass the assessment of evidence. Hence the GMC's decision to accept statements indicating satisfactory appraisal as evidence for revalidation. Where there is any doubt about a doctor's practice, there will be a full assessment, conducted by the GMC itself, using its performance procedures.

Mindful of the need to ensure a robust process, the GMC will therefore need to quality assure the process rigorously. In particular it will have to assure itself – and therefore the public – that proxy sources of evidence, such as employers' and peers' appraisals, are reliable. To this end it is intended to carry out random checks on the validity and reliability of the evidence offered by doctors from appraisal, and independently to seek information from patients and doctors' working colleagues who can give an insight into their practice. In this way collusion, inexperience or ineptness by the appraiser, or flaws in a local appraisal system, should be detected.

Fitness to practise

In cases where there are doubts about a doctor's fitness to practice, revalidation will feed into the existing Fitness to Practise procedures.

The new model will be divided into two stages, 'investigation' and 'adjudication'. These functions will both come within the ambit of the GMC but will be administered separately from each other and undertaken by different groups of people. The new model is a unitary system which will enable a doctor's fitness to practise to be considered in the round, whilst allowing that different methods will be required to deal with different aspects of dysfunctional practice.

The new procedures are based on the following principles. They must be:

- fair, objective, transparent and free from discrimination
- effective in protecting the public interest
- as prompt as is consistent with achieving fairness
- proportionate and consistent in process and outcome
- understandable to doctors and the general public

- compatible with the requirements of the European Convention of Human Rights (now incorporated into national law by the Human Rights Act 1998)
- an effective and distinct part of a wider framework for protecting patients, including measures taken by the NHS and other employers
- regarded with confidence by the public and the profession
- compatible with the view that the GMC's core role is to maintain the Medical Register.

Screening and investigation will be a single stage carried out under the supervision of the Investigation Committee of the Council. In investigating a complaint the task of the Committee will be to determine whether there is a more realistic prospect of establishing that the doctor's fitness to practise is impaired to a degree justifying action on registration. The Committee will be responsible for issuing warnings – another new development – in cases where there may be significant departures from *Good Medical Practice* which are not so serious as to justify restriction of the doctor's registration.

Adjudication will be carried out by medical and lay members of Fitness to Practise panels selected through open competitions against competencies. Members will be fully trained, regularly appraised and will have to show that they subscribe to GMC values and policies. The sanctions include no action (in exceptional cases only such as terminal illness), conditional registration, suspension and erasure. Panels will also have the power to issue a warning where there are significant departures from *General Medical Practice* not sufficient to affect registration. Warnings from the Investigation Committee or Fitness to Practise Panel will be fed into the processes of appraisal and revalidation. A separate Interim Orders Committee will continue, as now, to impose an interim order restricting or suspending a doctor's right to practise where the public interest requires this.

Three other general developments are worth mentioning here. First, all the processes will be quality assured at each stage against explicit operating standards. Many of those standards are already in use.

Second, as now the Council will prosecute the case, but no Council members will be involved in adjudication. So the Council, in bringing a case against a doctor, will be identified more positively in future as the guardian of the profession's standards.

Third, the GMC has accepted that, as part of its Fitness to Practise function, it will provide the kind of aggregate analysis of cases of the kind on which a start was made in, for example, cases of impaired clinical performance (2002) and in the evaluation of the health procedures in 1998.

What has emerged is no less than a radical rethink from first principles of the three historic procedures – conduct, health and performance – remodelled around a new concept of impaired fitness to practise in accordance with the principles of *Good Medical Practice*. The processes have been streamlined and incorporate modern concepts of fairness.

The changes in full

Appendix C contains a timeline showing the changes made in the regulation of doctors. This gives a full picture of what has been involved in the transformation of the old GMC into the new GMC.

References

1 Bristol Royal Infirmary Inquiry (2001) *Learning from Bristol: the report of the public inquiry into children's heart surgery at the Bristol Royal Infirmary, 1984–1995.* Stationery Office, London.

2 Smith R (1998) All changed, changed utterly. *BMJ.* **316**: 1917–18.

3 Calman K (1994) The profession of medicine. *BMJ.* **309**: 1140–3.

4 Shock M (1992) Medicine at the centre of the nation's affairs. *BMJ.* **309**: 1730–3.

5 Stacey M (1992) *Regulating British Medicine: the General Medical Council.* Wiley, Chichester.

6 Irvine DH (1997) The performance of doctors. I. Professionalism and regulation in a changing world. *BMJ.* **314**: 1540–2.

7 Irvine DH (1997) The performance of doctors. II. Maintaining good practice, protecting patients from poor performance. *BMJ.* **314**: 1613–15.

8 Stevens R (1966) *Medical Practice in Modern England: the impact of specialisation and state medicine.* Yale University Press, London.

9 Collings JS (1950) General practice in England today: a reconnaissance. *Lancet.* **1**: 555–85.

10 British Medical Association (1965) *A Charter for the Family Doctor Service.* BMA, London.

11 Coker N (2001) *Racism in Medicine: an agenda for change.* King's Fund, London.

12 Freidson E (1988) *Profession of Medicine: a study of the sociology of applied knowledge.* University of Chicago Press, London.

13 Stacey M (2000) The General Medical Council and self-regulation. In: D Gladstone (ed) *Regulating Doctors.* Institute for the Study of Civil Society, London.

14 Secretary of State for Social Services (1975) *Report of the Committee of Inquiry into the Regulation of the Medical Profession.* Chairman Dr AW Merrison. Cmnd 6018. Stationery Office, London.

15 Irvine DH (1999) The performance of doctors: the new professionalism. *Lancet.* **358**: 1174–7.

16 General Medical Council minutes, CX (1973), p. 179.

17   Pyke-Lees W (1958) *Centenary of the GMC 1858–1958: the history and present work of the Council.* GMC, London.

18   Richardson, Lord (1983) *The Council Transformed.* GMC Annual Report 1982. GMC, London.

19   Shaw B (1911) *The Doctor's Dilemma*, Act 1.

20   Shaw B (1957) *Preface to The Doctor's Dilemma.* Penguin, London.

21   Royal Commission on Medical Education (1968) *Report 1965–68.* Chairman Lord Todd. Cmnd 3569. Stationery Office, London.

22   Rivett G (1998) *From Cradle to Grave: fifty years of the NHS.* King's Fund, London.

23   Irvine DH (1972) *Teaching Practices.* Report from general practice No. 15. RCGP, London.

24   Royal College of General Practitioners (1972) *The Future General Practitioner: learning and teaching.* BMJ for RCGP, London.

25   Irvine DH (1975) *1984 – The Quiet Revolution.* William Pickles lecture, 1975. *J Roy Coll Gen Pract.* **25**: 599–604.

26   Royal College of General Practitioners (1985) *Evidence to the Royal Commission on the National Health Service 1977.* Republished by the College as Policy Statement 1. RCGP, London.

27   Royal College of General Practitioners (1974) Evidence to the inquiry into the regulation of the medical profession. *J Roy Coll Gen Pract.* **24**: 59–74.

28   Joseph, Sir Keith. *Hansard. House of Commons*, 23 November 1972, **846**, pp. 464–5.

29   Wells-Pestell, Lord. *Hansard. House of Lords.* **387**, p. 1166.

30   Report of a Committee of Enquiry set up for the Medical Profession in the United Kingdom (1976) *Competence to Practice.* Chairman Sir Anthony Alment. Published by the Committee.

31   General Medical Council (1987) *Recommendations on the Training of Specialists.* GMC, London.

32   Irvine DH (1983) Quality: our outstanding problem. *J Roy Coll Gen Pract.* **33**: 521–3.

33   Royal College of General Practitioners (1985) *Quality in General Practice.* Policy Statement No. 2. RCGP, London.

34   Royal College of General Practitioners (1985) *What Sort of Doctor?* Report from General Practice 23. RCGP, London.

35   Irvine DH, Russell IT, Hutchinson A *et al.* (1986) Educational development and evaluation in the Northern Region. In: D Pendleton, T Schofield and M Marinker (eds) *In Pursuit of Quality.* RCGP, London.

36   North of England Study of Standards and Performance in General Practice (1992) Medical audit in general practice. 1. Effects on doctors' clinical behaviour for common childhood conditions. *BMJ.* **304**: 1480–4.

37 North of England Study of Standards and Performance in General Practice (1992) Medical audit in general practice. 2. Effects on the health of patients with common childhood conditions. *BMJ.* **304**: 1484–8.

38 Kennedy I (1983) *The Unmasking of Medicine.* Granada, London.

39 Robinson J (1988) *A Patient's Voice at the GMC: a lay member's view of the General Medical Practice Council.* Health Rights, London.

40 Klein R (1983) *The Politics of the National Health Service.* Longman, London.

41 Smith R (1989) The day of judgement comes closer. *BMJ.* **298**: 1241–4.

42 Lock S (1989) Regulating doctors: a good case for the profession to set up a new inquiry. *BMJ.* **299**: 137–8.

43 Kilpatrick R (1989) Profiles of the GMC: portrait or caricature? *BMJ.* **299**: 109–12.

44 General Medical Council (1984) *Questions Concerning Serious Professional Misconduct – Working Party Report.* Council minutes, November 1984. Appendix XIX.

45 General Medical Council. Meeting of the Council, November 1984. Transcript of proceedings.

46 O'Donnell M (1986) A raw deal for all. *BMA News Review.* **Sept**: 41.

47 General Medical Council. Meeting of the Council, May 1987. Transcript of proceedings.

48 Secretaries of State for Health, England and Wales, Scotland and Northern Ireland (1989) *Working for Patients.* Cmnd 555. Stationery Office, London.

49 Department of Health (1990) *Medical Audit in the Family Practitioner Services.* Health circular. DoH, London.

50 Department of Health (1993) *Hospital Doctors: training for the future.* Report of the working group on specialist training. Chairman Kenneth Calman. DoH, London.

51 General Medical Council (1993) *Tomorrow's Doctors.* GMC, London.

52 General Medical Council (1995) *Good Medical Practice.* GMC, London.

53 Department of Health (1995) *Maintaining Medical Excellence: review of guidance on doctors' performance.* NHS Executive, London.

54 Donaldson L (1994) Doctors with problems in an NHS workforce. *BMJ.* **308**: 1277–82.

55 Rosenthal M (1995) *The Incompetent Doctor: behind closed doors.* Open University Press, Buckingham.

56 General Medical Council (2001) The General Medical Council's performance procedures: a study of their implementation and impact. Ed. Lesley Southgate. *Medical Education.* **35**: Supplement 1.

57 Smith R (1992) The GMC on performance: professional self-regulation is on the line. *BMJ.* **304**: 1257.

58   Smith R (1993) The end of the GMC? The government, not the GMC, is looking at under-performing doctors. *BMJ.* **307**: 954.

59   Irvine DH (2001) Doctors in the UK: their professionalism and its regulatory framework. *Lancet.* **358**: 1807–10.

60   Irvine DH (2001) The changing relationship between the public and the medical profession. *J Roy Soc Med.* **94**: 162–9.

61   Department of Health (1996) *A Service with Ambitions.* Stationery Office, London.

62   Department of Health (1997) *The New NHS: modern, dependable.* Stationery Office, London.

63   Department of Health (1998) *A First-class Service: quality in the NHS.* Stationary Office, London.

64   Department of Health (2000) *Building a Safer NHS for Patients.* DoH, London.

65   Department of Health (1999) *Supporting Doctors, Protecting Patients.* DoH, London.

66   Department of Health (2000) *The NHS Plan: a plan for investment, a plan for reform.* DoH, London.

67   Irvine DH and Donaldson L (1993) Quality and standards in health care. *Proc Roy Soc Edin.* **101B**: 1–30.

68   Allen I, Perkins E and Witherspoon S (1996) *The Handling of Complaints Against Doctors.* Report by Policy Studies Institute for the Racial Equality Group of the GMC. PSI, London.

69   Morgan M, White C and Fenwick N (1999) *An Evaluation of the General Medical Council's Health Procedures.* Nuffield Institute for Health, London.

70   General Medical Council Professional Conduct Committee, 17–18 June 2002. Transcript of proceedings.

71   Lords of the Judicial Committee of the Privy Council. *Dr John Roylance v The General Medical Council.* Privy Council appeal No. 49 of 1998, given on 24 March 1999.

72   Klein R (1998) Regulating the medical profession: doctors and the public interest. *Healthcare UK 1997/1998.* King's Fund, London.

73   General Medical Council (1998) *Good Medical Practice* (2e). GMC, London.

74   General Medical Council (1998) *Maintaining Good Medical Practice.* GMC, London.

75   McManus IC, Gordon D and Winder BC (2000) Duties of a doctor: UK doctors and *Good Medical Practice. Quality in Healthcare.* **9**: 14–22.

76   Hutchinson A, Williams M *et al.* (1999) Perceptions of *Good Medical Practice* in the NHS: a survey of senior health professionals. *Quality in Healthcare.* **8**: 213–18.

77   Ritchie J (2000) *The Report of the Inquiry into Quality and Practice with*

the NHS Arising from the Actions of Rodney Ledward. Stationery Office, London.

78 General Medical Council. Minutes of the meeting, November 1998.

79 Horton R (1998) UK medicine: what are we to do? *Lancet.* **352**: 1166.

80 General Medical Council. Internal Conference, February 1999. Transcript of proceedings.

81 General Medical Council. Minutes of the meeting of Council, February 1999.

82 The Shipman Inquiry (2002) *Death Disguised.* First Report Vol. 1. Chair Dame Janet Smith. Stationery Office, Norwich.

83 General Medical Council. Minutes of the meeting, 23 May 2000.

84 General Medical Council (2000) *Revalidating Doctors: ensuring standards, securing the future.* GMC, London.

85 General Medical Council (2001) *Effective, Inclusive and Accountable: reform of the GMC's structure, constitution and governance.* GMC, London.

86 General Medical Council (2001) *Acting Fairly to Protect Patients: reform of the GMC's Fitness to Practise procedures.* GMC, London.

87 General Medical Council (1998) *Seeking Patients' Consent: the ethical considerations.* GMC, London.

88 General Medical Council. Minutes of the meeting, May 2001.

89 Freidson E (1994) *Professionalism Reborn: theory, prophecy and policy.* Polity Press, Cambridge.

Appendix A: The duties of a doctor registered with the GMC

Patients must be able to trust doctors with their lives and well-being. To justify that trust, we as a profession have a duty to maintain a good standard of practice and care and to show respect for human life. In particular as a doctor you must:

- make the care of patients your first concern
- treat every patient politely and considerately
- respect patients' dignity and privacy
- listen to patients and respect their views
- give patients information in a way they can understand
- respect the rights of patients to be fully involved in decisions about their care
- keep your professional knowledge and skills up to date
- recognise the limits of your professional competence
- be honest and trustworthy
- respect and protect confidential information
- make sure that your personal beliefs do not prejudice your patients' care
- act quickly to protect patients from risk if you believe that you or a colleague may not be fit to practise
- avoid abusing your position as a doctor
- work with colleagues in the ways that best serve patients' interests.

Appendix B: The Bristol determination

THE CHAIRMAN: At the centre of this inquiry is the trust that patients place in their doctors. A parent placing a child in a doctor's care must have confidence that the doctor will put the child's best interests before any other. It is hard to imagine a situation in which trust is more essential. A doctor who fails to live up to that expectation will seriously undermine not only his or her relationship with that particular patient or parents, but the confidence of all patients in doctors.

This Committee must and will take action where it appears that a doctor has betrayed that trust. At the same time, we have not allowed emotion to distract us from our duty, which is to consider a charge against each of the doctors. Our duty is to be objective and fair.

In the course of the inquiry we have heard and read a massive quantity of evidence relating to the practice of two paediatric cardiac surgeons and the conduct of the Chief Executive at the Bristol Royal Infirmary. That evidence has come from parents, from doctors and other staff at the hospital, from experts and others.

We have taken the utmost care to avoid judging the doctors with the benefit of hindsight. We have kept firmly in mind that the most conscientious of doctors can, and do, make mistakes. People rightly expect high standards of doctors; but we must not judge doctors mercilessly according to the highest achievable performance. To do so would make medical practice impossible and would be contrary to the interests of patients.

In considering all our findings of fact and our findings of serious professional misconduct, we have applied the standard of proof required by law.

Mr Wisheart, patients and their families were entitled to expect that, as a registered medical practitioner, as a consultant, as an associate clinical director and as a medical director, you would comply with proper professional standards. You failed to do so in three main ways.

First, you carried out the last three AVSD operations referred to in Schedule B when 50 per cent of the patients in the preceding 12 operations had died. The causes of death varied considerably. The Committee have heard that you 'wrestled' in your mind with the high mortality rate, which was substantially higher than the published figures for hospitals elsewhere. 'Wrestling' was not enough. You knew that Mr Dhasmana was achieving much better results for the same operation in the same hospital, but you took no adequate steps to establish the causes of this difference. You were aware of the concerns of colleagues. You justified the continuation of your AVSD programme by pointing to the particular difficulties which arose in a number of the operations which you undertook.

The Committee accepts that during the course of your AVSD series you encountered a number of patients with particularly complex problems. Having carefully considered the expert evidence, we have concluded that after the twelfth AVSD operation you should have stopped to undertake a review, involving others, of your AVSD operations. You should have sought adequate retraining, assistance or advice. You should have resumed this type of operation only if colleagues who had reviewed your previous results had advised that it was safe for you to do so. Your decision to continue to operate in the absence of such an independent review was a serious departure from safe professional standards.

Second, the information about mortality rates which you gave to the mother of Matthew Rundle and the parents of Hanna Silcox was misleading. You advised Mrs Rundle that the AVSD operation on her son had a 20 to 25 per cent risk of mortality. You advised the parents of Hanna Silcox that the same operation on their daughter had about a 20 per cent risk of mortality. You gave your advice on the basis of your knowledge of published mortality rates, your assessment of the problems you had encountered in your recent operations and your assessment of the operation about which you were giving advice. However, at the time when you gave this advice your own observed mortality rate for this operation was 50 per cent. You did not tell the parents this, nor give them a basis for comparison. In this way, you denied the parents the facts they needed in order to make informed decisions about their children's treatment. You left the parents with a misleadingly optimistic impression of the prospects of successful outcomes.

Third, by the time of the operation on Joshua Loveday you were, by your own admission, aware of general concerns about Mr Dhasmana's switch operations. In the two days prior to this operation concerns were specifically expressed to you as medical director about the operation proceeding. Professor Angelini informed you in writing that he would dissociate himself from the consequences if the operation went ahead.

You decided with Dr Roylance that an external review was necessary. At the meeting on 11 January 1995, which you convened and chaired, it was your professional duty to inform the meeting, and in particular Mr Dhasmana, of this critical information. You also failed to satisfy yourself that an up-to-date assessment of the patient's condition was available to enable the meeting to consider whether an operation on the next day was necessary. As a result, the meeting – in the absence of crucial information – agreed that the operation should be undertaken by Mr Dhasmana the next morning when this was not in Joshua Loveday's best interests.

The Committee has concluded that in these three respects you fell seriously short of proper professional standards. We should make it clear that we have not taken into account our findings of fact under head 6 in reaching our determinations under rules 29, 30 and 31. These findings under head 6 do not, in all the circumstances, add to your culpability.

The Committee has judged you to have been guilty of serious professional misconduct in relation to the facts found proved against you in the charge. We have considered very carefully the extensive evidence of the care and dedication which you have shown to many patients. We accept that over many years you have worked hard in their service. We also accept that there is no evidence that you ever had any intention of acting other than in your patients' interests. Those facts make the need for this inquiry all the more tragic. We have noted your intention not to resume practice.

The Committee has concluded that, given the gravity of the matters proved against you, and these mitigating factors notwithstanding, it is necessary in the public interest to direct the Registrar to erase your name from the Register.

Unless you exercise your right of appeal, your name will be erased from the Register 28 days from today. That concludes your case.

Mr Dhasmana, the Committee accepts the evidence of Mr Brawn that in view of your experience with non-neonates you were entitled to start a programme of operations for transposition of the great arteries in neonates. The Committee also accepts that you were entitled to continue with this programme until after the operation on Thomas Pottage on 13 July 1993. Following his death, you properly recognised that your results were such that you should not continue to perform these operations unless and until you had identified and corrected the cause of your excessive mortality.

Moreover, the Committee has noted the steps which you took to discuss your mortality figures with others and your attempts to improve your skills by visiting Mr Brawn at Birmingham on two occasions. You made changes to your practice as a result of the first visit. It is clear that you made some effort – though an insufficient one – to address the problems which you were recognising. You were concerned enough to do this.

Nonetheless, your mortality rate for neonatal arterial switch operations continued to be very poor throughout the period in question. When you returned from Birmingham after your second visit in July 1993 you still had not, according to your own evidence, established the cause of your poor results. You could not, therefore, resume the programme safely. You told us that you thought you needed more experience. In those circumstances, your decision to resume operating on neonates was, in the Committee's view, a serious departure from safe and proper practice.

It is for that reason that the Committee decided that patient D33 should be the first patient in Schedule D to the charge. It is irrelevant to this conclusion that the first operation after your return from Birmingham was in fact successful. In the judgment of the Committee you should not have carried out this operation at all. The second, on Niall McKelvey, was not successful and it was only then that, belatedly, you decided finally to cease arterial switch operations on neonates.

You faced a dilemma in connection with the operation on Joshua Loveday. Your colleagues in the paediatric cardiac unit, other than Dr Bolsin, were united in their view that on clinical grounds there was no reason for you to refrain from carrying out this operation. However, you were aware that colleagues were expressing concerns about paediatric cardiac surgery in general and this proposed operation in particular. Moreover, you knew or ought to have known that your results in arterial switch operations on non-neonates were less satisfactory than those achieved in other centres.

The decision to operate was finally your responsibility. You should have satisfied yourself about the immediate clinical condition of Joshua, in particular whether there was such a degree of urgency that the surgery had to be performed at Bristol the next day. It is the judgment of the Committee that you should have concluded that Joshua Loveday's interests would not be best served by operating on him on 12 January 1995. In deciding to operate, you failed in your duty to the patient and his parents.

The Committee has judged you to have been guilty of serious professional misconduct in relation to the facts proved against you in the charge. We have carefully considered the evidence of the dedication and care which you have shown to patients. We have also taken into account the evidence that you took steps, albeit insufficient ones, to address the problems which you were facing. Furthermore, when you decided to operate on Joshua Loveday, Mr Wisheart and Dr Roylance had denied you crucial information. In all these circumstances we have directed that for a period of three years your registration shall be conditional on your compliance with the following requirement: you shall not undertake paediatric cardiac surgery.

Unless you exercise your right of appeal, your registration will become subject to the specified conditions 28 days after the date when written notice of the direction is deemed to have been served upon you.

The Committee will resume consideration of your case at a meeting to be held before the end of the three-year period. They will then consider whether to take further action in relation to your registration. You will be informed of the date of that meeting, which you will be expected to attend. Shortly before the resumed hearing you will be asked to supply the Council with the names of professional colleagues and other persons to whom the Council may apply for information as to their knowledge of your conduct throughout the interval since this hearing of your case.

That concludes your case.

Dr Roylance, now and at the times referred to in the charge you were a registered medical practitioner. It is as a registered medical practitioner that the Committee has judged you in respect of all the findings of fact.

The Committee accepts that chief executives, whether medically qualified or not, cannot and should not attempt to intervene in the day-to-day clinical decisions of their medical colleagues. Registered medical practitioners who are chief executives have nonetheless a clear responsibility to intervene wherever necessary to ensure the safety of patients.

The public expects members of the medical profession to put patients' needs first. This applies not only in the consulting room and the operating theatre, but in other areas where doctors' actions or inactions may affect the welfare of patients.

As Chief Executive of the United Bristol Healthcare NHS Trust (and previously as district general manager) from 1990 to 1994, you were made aware that senior medical colleagues of yours had serious concerns about excessive mortality of patients undergoing paediatric cardiac surgery. These concerns are specified in the findings of fact and included the letter of 21 July 1994 from Dr Doyle, the contents of which were known to you. As Chief Executive, you were in a position to enquire into those concerns, to find out whether they were justified or not and, if necessary, to intervene. As a medical practitioner registered with this Council you had a duty to act to protect patients from harm.

Your own evidence demonstrates that you chose, over a long period, to ignore the concerns which were being brought to your attention, preferring to leave these matters to the consultants concerned. Yet, faced with information suggesting that children were being placed at unnecessary risk, you took no adequate steps to establish the truth. You knew that your medical director was at the centre of many of these concerns, yet you took no adequate steps to obtain impartial advice from appropriate specialists.

In the case of Joshua Loveday, you knew that his operation was scheduled to take place against a background of serious concerns, over a prolonged period, about the performance of complex paediatric cardiac surgery including switch operations at the BRI. You were approached by Professor Angelini and Dr Doyle from the Department of Health, both of whom urged you not to let the operation go ahead. In response to such concerns, you decided with Mr Wisheart that an external review was necessary. Despite that, without taking appropriate external advice, without making independent enquiries of your own, and without exploring alternatives for safeguarding Joshua Loveday's interests, you took no steps to prevent the operation from proceeding. By your failure to take adequate action, you failed to safeguard Joshua Loveday's proper interests.

The Committee has judged you to have been guilty of serious professional misconduct in relation to the facts proved against you in the charge. We have considered very carefully the evidence of your contributions to the Health Service over a long period. That makes the need for this inquiry all the more tragic. We have noted that you have retired.

Nonetheless, the Committee has concluded that, given the gravity of the matters proved against you, it is necessary in the public interest to direct the Registrar to erase your name from the Register.

Unless you exercise your right of appeal, your name will be erased from the Register 28 days from today. That concludes your case.

Having concluded our determinations in respect of the three doctors, the Committee wishes to identify a number of issues which arose during the course of the inquiry. These wider issues concern the practice of surgery and of medicine generally, and will have to be addressed by the medical profession. The issues include:

- the need for clearly understood clinical standards
- how clinical competence and technical expertise are assessed and evaluated
- who carries the responsibility in team-based care
- the training of doctors in advanced procedures
- how to approach the so-called learning curve of doctors undertaking established procedures
- the reliability and validity of the data used to monitor doctors' personal performance

- the use of medical and clinical audit
- the appreciation of the importance of factors, other than purely clinical ones, that can affect clinical judgement, performance and outcome
- the responsibility of a consultant to take appropriate actions in response to concerns about his or her performance
- the factors which appear to discourage openness and frankness about doctors' personal performance
- how doctors explain risks to patients
- the ways in which people concerned about patient safety can make their concerns known
- the need for doctors to take prompt action at an early stage where a colleague is in difficulty, in order to offer the best chance of avoiding damage to patients and the colleague, and of putting things right.

We have in addition been concerned by the evidence suggesting institutional failures at the BRI and beyond.

These matters cannot be addressed by an inquiry of this kind but clearly need to be addressed urgently by the profession and others.

Copies of this announcement will now be made available.

That concludes the hearing.

Appendix C: Timeline of the GMC reforms

GMC

External events

1975: The Merrison Report

1976: Alment Committee on Competence to Practise

1978: Medical Act 1978, establishing health procedures

1982: Sir John Walton elected President

1983: Dr Arthur Archer appeared before PCC

1984: Nigel Spearing's Private Member's Bill

1987–89: Working Party on competence issues

1989: Sir Robert Kilpatrick elected President

1990: Working Party on arrangements to deal with seriously deficient performance

1990: New contract for GPs

1993: *Tomorrow's Doctors* published

1995: First edition of *Good Medical Practice* published

1995 (Jan): Joshua Loveday died

1995: Medical (Professional Performance) Act, establishing performance procedures

1995: Sir Donald Irvine elected
President

1996–98: GMC inquiries into
Bristol doctors

1996: Local inquiry into Rodney
Ledward

1998 (May): Council approves new
edition of *GMP*, explicitly linking
standards with registration

1998 (June): Conclusion of Bristol
case at the PCC

1998 (June): 'Dear Roddy' letter

1998 (September): Rodney
Ledward erased by the PCC

1998 (November): Council
discusses revalidation for the first
time

1999 (February): Council
conference about revalidation
(agreement to link with
registration and coverage of all
doctors)

1999 (March): Roylance Appeal
dismissed by Lords

1999 (September): Harold Shipman
arrested and charged with murder

1999 (September): Government
published *Supporting Doctors,
Protecting Patients*

2000 (31 January): Harold Shipman
convicted of 15 murders

2000 (11 February): Harold
Shipman erased by PCC

2000 (February): critical BMA
Council meeting

2000 (May): Council agreed to
consult on revalidation; agreed
new interim orders process; agreed
to appoint external people to
PCC; agreed principles for new
constitution

2000 (June): Launch of consultation on revalidation

2000 (June) report of NHS Inquiry into Rodney Ledward (Chair: Miss Jean Ritchie QC)

2000 (June): BMA Senior Hospital Doctors Conference vote of no confidence in currently constituted GMC; Academy of Medical Royal Colleges suspends its membership of Joint Consultants' Committee and disassociates itself from the motion

2000 (July) BMA Representative Meeting vote of no confidence in currently constituted GMC

2000 (July): Richard Neale erased by PCC

2000 (July): Special conference on governance and Fitness to Practise reform

2000 (July): Report of Bristol Inquiry (Chair: Professor Sir Ian Kennedy)

2000 (July): Medical Act (Amendment) Order, establishing Interim Orders Committee, longer minimum period before restoration of erased doctors and outside members of Conduct Committee

2001 (January): Alder Hey Report (retention of organs without consent)

2001 (February): Council agreed principles of new Fitness to Practise procedures

2001 (April): meeting with BMA and Academy about constitution of GMC

2001 (May): Council decides to seek legislation on revalidation

2001 (June): stakeholder
conference: agreement on size and
constitution of new Council

2001 (November): conclusion of
consultation on constitution of
Council; agreement on design of
new Fitness to Practise procedures;
Sir Graeme Catto elected President

2002 (May): Government
published draft order
implementing GMC's reform
proposals

2002 (December): Medical Act
(Amendment) Order approved,
enabling introduction of
revalidation, new Fitness to
Practise procedures and new,
smaller Council

Glossary 1: The principal players

Alberti, Professor Sir George
President, Royal College of Physicians of London, 1997–2002; GMC, 1999–present

Allen, Dr Isobel
Researcher and analyst, Policy Studies Institute; produced reports on allegations of discrimination in GMC's Fitness to Practise Committees

Alment, Sir Anthony
Past President of Royal College of Obstetricians; Chair, Enquiry into Competence to Practise

Bogle, Dr Ian
Chair of the General Medical Services Committee of the BMA, 1997–99; Chair of Council of the BMA, 1997–present

Borman, Edwin
Member of BMA Central Consultants' and Specialists' Committee, 1996–present; GMC, 1994–present

Calman, Sir Kenneth
Chief Medical Officer for England, 1991–98

Chantler, Professor Sir Cyril
Chair, Council of Heads of UK Medical Schools, 1998–99; Chair, GMC Standards Committee, 1997–2003

Chisholm, Dr John
Chair of General Medical Services Committee of BMA, 1997–present; GMC, 1999–present

Clarke, Kenneth
Secretary of State for Health, 1988–90

Dobson, Frank
Secretary of State for Health, 1997–99

Donaldson, Professor Sir Liam
Chief Medical Officer for England, 1998–present

Grabham, Sir Anthony
BMA Council, 1975–present; current BMA President; GMC, 1979–99

Gray, Professor Sir Denis Pereira
President of the RCGP, 1997–2000; Chair of the Academy of Medical Royal Colleges, 2000–02; GMC, 1994–present

Hawker, Peter
Chair of BMA Central Consultants' and Specialists' Committee, 1998–2002

Hine, Dame Deirdre
Formerly, CMO Wales; Chair of CHI, 1999–present

Horton, Richard
Editor of the *Lancet*

Jackson, Sir Barry
President, Royal College of Surgeons of England, 1998–2001; GMC, 1999–present

Johnson, James
Chair, BMA Central Consultants' and Specialists' Committee, 1994–98; Chair, Joint Consultants' Committee, 1998–present

Kennedy, Sir Ian
GMC member, 1984–93; Chair of the Bristol Inquiry, 2001; Chair designate of CHAI

Kilpatrick, Sir Robert (now Lord)
President of GMC, 1989–94

Klein, Professor Rudolf
Professor of Social Policy, University of Bath, 1978–96

Langlands, Sir Alan
Chief Executive of NHS, 1994–2000

Macara, Sir Alexander
Chair of Council at BMA, 1993–98; GMC, 1979–2002

MacSween, Sir Roderick
President of Royal College of Pathologists, 1996–99; Chair of Academy of Medical Royal Colleges, 1999–2000; GMC, 1999–present

Merrison, Sir Alec
Nuclear physicist; past Vice-chancellor of Bristol University; Chair of Merrison Committee, 1975

Milburn, Alan
Minister of State for Health, 1997–98; Secretary of State for Health, 1999–present

Pringle, Professor Mike
Chair of RCGP, 1998–2001

Robinson, Jean
Lay member of GMC, 1979–93

Scott, Finlay
Registrar; Chief Executive of GMC, 1994–present

Shaw, Professor David
Dean of Medicine, University of Newcastle, 1981–89; Chair of GMC Education Committee, 1989–94

Smith, Richard
Editor, *British Medical Journal*

Southgate, Professor Dame Lesley
GMC Lead on developing performance procedures, 1994–present; President of RCGP, 2000–03

Spearing, Nigel MP
Raised the case of Alfie Winn and the meaning of serious professional misconduct

Stacey, Professor Margaret
Lately, Professor of Medical Sociology, University of Warwick; GMC lay member, 1976–84

Walton, Sir John (now Lord)
President of GMC, 1982–89

Wells, Sir William
Chair, NHS South Thames RHA and later South East Region, 1994–2001; Chair of NHS Appointments Commission, 2001–present

Glossary 2: The key institutions

Academy of Royal Medical Colleges and Faculties (The Academy)
Action for the Victims of Medical Accidents (AVMA)
The Audit Comission
British Medical Association (BMA)
College of Health
Commission for Health Audit and Inspection (CHAI)
Commission for Health Improvement (CHI)
Commission for Patient and Public Involvement in Health
Community Health Councils (CHCs)
Consumers' Association (CA)
Council for the Regulation of Health Care Professionals (CRHP)
Department of Health (England and Wales) (DoH)
General Medical Council (GMC)
General Medical Services Committee (GMSC) of the BMA, now the
  General Practitioners' Committee (GPC)
Joint Committee on Postgraduate Training for General Practice
  (JCPTGP)
Joint Consultants' Committee (JCC)
National Clinical Assessment Authority (NCAA)
National Health Service (NHS)
National Institute for Clinical Excellence (NICE)
National Patient Safety Agency (NPSA)
Overseas Doctors' Association (ODA)
Patients' Association
Postgraduate Medical Education and Training Board (PMETB)
Professional Conduct Committee (PCC) of the GMC
Royal College of Anaesthetists
Royal College of General Practitioners (RCGP)
Royal College of Nursing (RCN)

Royal College of Obstetricians and Gynaecologists (RCOG)
Royal College of Physicians of Edinburgh (RCP Edinburgh)
Royal College of Physicians of London (RCP)
Royal College of Surgeons of Edinburgh (RCS Edinburgh)
Royal College of Surgeons of England (RCS)
Royal Society of Medicine (RSM)
The Society of Cardiothoracic Surgeons of Great Britain and Ireland
Specialist Training Authority (STA)
United Kingdom Council for Nursing, Midwifery and Health Visiting
   (UKCC) – replaced by the Nursing and Midwifery Council

Index